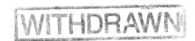

Working and Caring for a Child with Chronic Illness

Working and Caring for a Child with Chronic Illness

Disconnected and Doing it All

Margaret H. Vickers
University of Western Sydney

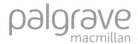

First published 2006 by
PALGRAVE MACMILLAN
Houndmills, Basingstoke, Hampshire RG21 6XS and
175 Fifth Avenue, New York, N.Y. 10010
Companies and representatives throughout the world

PALGRAVE MACMILLAN is the global academic imprint of the Palgrave Macmillan division of St. Martin's Press, LLC and of Palgrave Macmillan Ltd. Macmillan® is a registered trademark in the United States, United Kingdom and other countries. Palgrave is a registered trademark in the European Union and other countries.

ISBN-13: 978–1–4039–9767–8   hardback
ISBN-10: 1–4039–9767–5   hardback

This book is printed on paper suitable for recycling and made from fully managed and sustained forest sources.

A catalogue record for this book is available from the British Library.

Library of Congress Cataloging-in-Publication Data
Vickers, Margaret H. (Margaret Heather), 1962–
    Working and caring for a child with chronic illness : disconnected and doing it all / by Margaret H. Vickers.
        p. cm.
    Includes bibliographical references and index.
    ISBN 1–4039–9767–5 (cloth)
        1. Chronically ill children–Medical care. 2. Chronically ill children–Care. 3. Sick children–Care. I. Title.

RJ380.V552 2006
618.92–dc22   2005056597

10   9   8   7   6   5   4   3   2   1
15   14   13   12   11   10   09   08   07   06

Printed and bound in Great Britain by
Antony Rowe Ltd, Chippenham and Eastbourne

To Michael: Being with you makes all things possible

Contents

Acknowledgements

I would like to formally acknowledge the contribution of the nine women who participated in this study. Without their preparedness to share, this book would not have been possible.

Financial support is also gratefully acknowledged from the Children's Hospital Education Research Institute (CHERI), Trauma Research International Pty Ltd, and the University of Western Sydney.

Part I
A Problem in the Spotlight

Prologue

Their Story: 'No-one ever asked about *me* before...'

This book is about *their story*, the story of the lives of women who cared for a child with a significant chronic illness or disability. I remember when I first met Evalyn. I was a little nervous; I wondered if she was too. I asked her, before we started our interview, how she felt. I was surprised by her answer. While Evalyn did confirm that she was also a little nervous, she was also 'a little bit excited' about our meeting: 'No one has ever asked about *me* before', she said. Dolly reported a similar experience:

Researcher: Thinking back to the last session we had, how did you feel after the last session?

Dolly: I found it quite cathartic actually, because you don't actually get to speak to many people about the honesty of the reality that you live in. People don't usually want to hear what it's really like (Dolly, Interview 2: 1; Vickers and Parris, 2005: 104).

I asked myself again: did I really want to interfere in these people's lives? Would I be able to do justice to what they shared so candidly? And would I be able to live with the consequences of my encounters and their outcomes (Bar-On, 1996: 9)?

Far from wondering if I can live with them, I feel uplifted by them; honoured that these women (yes, they were all women; more about that later) were prepared to share so much of themselves and their lives. And these were *great* women! Forthright, good-humoured, reflective, strong, capable and independent. I thoroughly enjoyed meeting them, talking with them, sharing their fears, tears and laughter.

This research journey began, as many do, serendipitously. I have no children myself, and yet here I was launching a research project that asked parents about their experiences. Most of my past research had been about things I had lived. I had written as a complete insider to the phenomenon at hand. Not this time. And I was nervous. Would I be able to relate to their parenting concerns when I had no children of my own?

However, it was the result of discussions with a colleague,[1] who had done much work in the area of childhood chronic illness and disability, and in children's special education, that I first recognised the potential contribution that *my* past research experience might have. I had completed much storied research work about adults with chronic illness and disability, exploring their journey through life and work as it related to their illness and disability. While I knew nothing about children, I reminded myself again, this was *not* a study about children; lots had already been done on *their* experiences with illness and disability. This study was about parents *who combined working and caring*. It felt like much of my previous work had brought me to this place. So I set out to find out: what was life like, working and caring for a child with a chronic illness? Was it a problem? I thought it likely. And so it began.

These women had the most amazing stories to share. The thing that hit me 'between the eyes' was that several of them told me that this was the first time that anyone had sat down *with them* and asked about *their* story, *their* concerns, *their* fears – what *they* thought and felt. For once, the person asking the questions was not asking about how their child was doing; how their child's illness was progressing or improving; how their child was doing at school; whether they were relating well to others or, more generally, if their child was coping with life. I asked, instead, how *the parents* felt; what *they* thought; how *they* responded to what life had presented them. I trust I have done their stories justice and feel pleased that the wheel is now turning towards further work to assist and support them.[2]

The interviews were not always easy. When asked, after the interview, how they had found the experience of sharing such harrowing episodes, many respondents shrugged, indicating that their participation had not really been a problem. As we saw earlier, some had even found it a distinctly positive experience. However, I also believed that some may not have enjoyed what had been awakened in them, having been deeply affected by what they had lived. The sharing and reflections that flowed as a result of this research might have shifted their lives in a material and not altogether comfortable fashion.

I didn't shrug. It was tough. As their tears flowed, tears pricked my own eyes. I had to work *very* hard to remain composed as I gathered their thoughts, their pain and their frustrations. I tried to remain the professional researcher: concerned, empathic and interested. This wasn't an act: their stories moved me; stories of betrayal, cruelty, hurt, grief, fear, loss, lack of support, being alone, feeling overwhelmed – and of being *so tired*. But still they all kept going. I don't know how. I admired them, tremendously. While writing this book, I also engaged with what they experienced, deliberately eschewing the neutral place of 'researcher' to better share what I had learned.

I cannot thank the participants in this study enough. Not only did they find time – around everything else – for this research, with its endless questions, constructed vignettes and lengthy discussions, they did so with charm, patience and grace. They also managed to do all this in between working full-time and caring for a child with a chronic illness. As readers will see, this was no small feat. I am touched. I am grateful. I am honoured.

To all those fabulous (unnamed) women – thank you. I hope this helps.

Introduction

Dear Diary

I awake this morning, about 5.30 am, with a start. The alarm shocks me into consciousness. That's unusual. Starting the day is never easy, but on this particular morning the piercing beeps slap me awake with about as much sensitivity as a Mack truck. I drag myself out from under the warm covers, moving towards my son David's room, as is my first-thing-to-do-every-day habit. David is stirring – but not much. I wonder why he has stayed so quiet on this particular morning. He is usually wide awake by now – far more ready for the day than I ever am. He has usually 'helped' me awake well before the alarm jettisons my dreams. His lassitude is unlikely to be a courtesy to me after such a rough night. In so many ways, David is such a lovely child, but his radar for my needs is not finely tuned.

Last night was hell. On my own these days, I have to tackle all that David unwittingly throws my way. And I have to do it all by myself. My partner, Jack, and I separated about six months ago. He had become increasingly distant towards me, and increasingly frustrated by David, in particular, David's developmental progress, or lack thereof. I think that, deep down, Jack was very disappointed in David. Perhaps he blames me? I don't know. We never really talked about it. What I do know is that once David was born, the bottom dropped out of our lives. Nothing was ever the same for either of us. Parenting a child with an intellectual disability left us little time or energy for the luxury of long, intellectual or emotional musings on how each of us might feel, what each of us might want from life, or what might lie ahead. Jack's response to the situation was to find comfort in the arms of another. That hurt.

As thoughts of David's future leap to the fore yet again, I wonder, what will happen to him when Jack and I are gone from this earth? Who will care for him? I have no idea. Daily life, for me at least, has become a daily battle of attrition: protracted, without victor, and completely exhausting and dispiriting for all involved. I just get through the day as best I can. Along the way, there has been much pain, many new experiences, and scars left in each of us that are hard to define, sometimes acutely sensitised and painful. I am reminded of a Vietnam veteran's scars of war: difficult to talk about, and impossible for those around to see or truly understand. That said, there has been much joy in my son too. It's just that I rarely have a moment – or the energy – to think about the good stuff.

I check David more closely and find him lethargic and irritable. While David does not talk, I have learned the signs and, especially, to sense immediately when all is not well. All is not well this morning. I note David's flushed face and feel his overly warm forehead with my hand. He has a temperature. This is not good. What to do? I find a thermometer tucked close at hand in a drawer. His temperature is high; I think it is too high for me to try and lower it with a cool bath and some Panadol. As I take this in, I look despairingly at David's soiled sheets and pyjamas: David is not toilet trained and, today, when he is obviously also unwell, contemplating this requires a couple of deep breaths to control my rising panic. Some days (this is one of them) I feel as though I am hanging on by my fingernails. Another deep breath – I remind myself that there is, simply, no-one else. Get over it.

My mind races; I consider my next move. A high temperature can be dangerous for any child and certainly explains his wakeful and unhappy night last night. David had awakened several times during the night, squealing and crying. The last time he woke, it took me well over an hour to settle him down. I did not notice if he had a temperature during the night. While trying to get David back to sleep, I was thinking of my client presentation scheduled this morning at nine o'clock. Ahhh! I remember it now and feel even more overwhelmed than before. All I could think about last night was David going back to sleep so I could too.

Now I feel guilty. While I was busy wondering how on earth I was going to function today, without any sleep, my son might have needed medical care. Now, what is important is getting David some help. I resolve to take him to the emergency room at the local hospital, rather than wait for the doctor's surgery to open for business at 9.00 am. While our doctor is pretty good at seeing David quickly when it is an emergency, with a fever like this, I don't want to wait.

I clean up David quickly – the bedclothes will have to wait – and take the opportunity to sponge him down to cool him off. I dress him in clean pyjamas and, as he crawls around the floor rather lethargically, I throw on some clothes myself. There is no time for a shower or anything else. I bundle David into the car, and head for the hospital. By now, it is about 6.00 am.

I arrive at the emergency room at the hospital. It is midweek and early in the morning. Good, there are not many others ahead of me. The triage nurse examines David, takes a brief history, and asks me to fill out the standard forms (which I do while holding on to David's squirming presence at the same time – not easy). When all that is done, I settle to wait for a doctor to see us.

I ring Jack on my mobile. His vaguely irritated and sleepy voice answers. I have his full attention when I tell him where I am and what is happening. He volunteers to come down to the hospital straight away, but then remembers he has an important appointment scheduled at 8.30 am that he really doesn't want to miss. Can I handle things there? Will the doctor be long? Should he come down anyway? What should he do? It is my turn to be irritated as I tell him that everything that can be done is being done, but to leave his phone on. I promise to call him after we have seen the doctor and let him know what is happening.

What now??

First, I call David's carer. While I usually take the 'morning shift', getting David ready for school and onto the bus that takes him to his special school, I hire a carer to handle the 'afternoon shift', the period in the afternoon when I am still working and David has finished school. Mary, David's current carer and the person I rely on the most, has been quite good. She is reliable, pleasant, and handles David with a great level of comfort (if, maybe, a little too carefree sometimes?). I also trust having her in my home when I am not there. However, she is almost finished university. What will happen then, when she will presumably want to pursue her own hard-won career? I block that out of my mind. She is one in a long line of carers that I have employed over the years, since David was born and I returned to work; some good, many not-so-good; all hard to find.

As I speak with Mary, I tell her that, depending on what happens when David sees the doctor, the day might shape up differently than planned. Can she come earlier than 3 pm to look after him if needed? I explain that I would very much like to get to the office at some point to at least try and repair some of the damage that is seemingly unavoidable at this stage. No, she can't, unfortunately. She has a test today, and can only come at 3 o'clock, as arranged. Shit!

It is now 7 am. I need to make the necessary calls to cancel that early morning presentation. What to do? I rifle through my phone book to see if, perchance, I have the mobile number of the client. I don't. I call my colleague, also involved in the planned presentation, and who knows the client. I ask her (beg her) to please call the client and alert her to my situation. She checks her phone book: she doesn't have the client's mobile number either. My heart sinks. She assures me that she is almost ready to leave home anyway and will make the call just as soon as she arrives at the office. Unfortunately, while she does this as promised, by the time she gets to the office and makes the call, the client is already making her way from her car, parked in our building, to our scheduled appointment. Too late! My colleague apologises to the client, profusely, explaining the emergency with my son. I also ring the client later that day and do the same. She says she understands; that 'these things happen'. I idly wonder though, given the tone of her voice, whether this might have dampened her enthusiasm to work with me in the future. No time to think about that now. I have done what I could to avoid inconveniencing anyone. That is, simply, the best I can do. The doctor calls our name and I gratefully take David in to see him.

The doctor examines David. I have mixed feelings right now: guilt, worry, frustration, and exhaustion. When David and I leave the doctor, with instructions for David's care, I find that Jack is in the waiting room, looking smooth, fresh and unruffled. Luckily, I am able to tell him that, according to the doctor, David appears just to have a touch of the flu and an inflamed throat. The doctor has instructed me to do the usual things to lower David's temperature and, of course, to keep a close eye on him. If there is any worsening of his condition, I am to consult my family doctor, or return to the emergency department, immediately.

By now, of course, I feel (and, no doubt, look) a wreck. Jack has clearly taken time to shower, have his breakfast and ready himself for work. For all my irritation, I know Jack loves David – a lot – and he worries when he is unwell. It's just that he doesn't seem to allow his concerns to interrupt his life in the same way I seem to find mine interrupted. He explains that he 'had to' get ready for work before coming in, because he had an important presentation to make to a client this morning and wouldn't have had time to go home and change if he had come straight here. I find myself grinding my teeth. Besides, he reminds me, I was already at the hospital where all the right people were doing everything that could be done. There was nothing he could have done to expedite the situation. And, besides, David just has a cold! Wasn't that lucky? I say nothing. I thank Jack for coming over and remind him of the time so he doesn't miss his appointment. There seems no point in both of us missing out on valuable income.

However, I feel foolish now, as well as irritated. While David is unwell and has a virus and a sore throat, this wasn't really an emergency situation.

My day is trashed. I call David's school first to tell them that he won't be in for the next few days. I call my mother and beg her to help me out – again. I explain that Mary will be over at 3.00 pm but can she come earlier? She is not very interested in caring for David today. Actually, since we had a serious quarrel a few months ago, she hasn't been very interested in caring for David at all. She tells me – again – that she has a life too, and plans, and friends, and things to do. She has done her share of child minding and working over the years and wants some time for herself to be with her friends. She finally agrees, grudgingly reminding me that she will have to cancel her bridge day, for the fourth time this year. She also reminds me, again, that I really need to find another person to be on standby to look after David when it is needed. I know she is right; I just haven't had the time to pursue it.

I take David home, make sure he can't come to any harm, put on the wash, and jump in the shower. As I stand there, with the warm water running over me, I feel completely overwhelmed. I have today covered, but what about tomorrow? What about my client? What will they think of me at work? I start to cry. I cry and cry. It is a long shower.

I finally get out of the shower, dress quickly, dry my hair and do my best to cover up the blotchy, puffy outcome of all those tears. My mother will be here soon. At least I should be able to get in to the office by around 11 or 12. Not a completely lost day.

As for tomorrow, I will call Kerry and see if she is still available…

This diary entry is fiction. However, its value lies in the fact that it has been constructed from the accounts of numerous women who have lived the phenomenon under review (Vallant, 2005). On that basis, I believe the diary entry to be a reasoned representation of a day in the life of a full-time working parent of a child with chronic illness. Please don't be fooled into thinking that this kind of day could never happen. It has been generated using a combination of the many experiences that were shared in this study. While no individual had lived this particular day, many of them reported days that were just like it. It is representative of their life experiences and the challenges, fears and uncertainty they routinely faced. I developed this fictional diary entry to give readers a glimpse into what life might be like for these people;

to put themselves in the frame; to think about how they might think and feel, and how they might react under similar circumstances.

However, throughout this volume, the narratives shared *are* the actual reflections, musings, contemplations, feelings and meanings of the respondents who participated. They are based on a very sharp reality. The stories are of lives that are real – sometimes painfully so – and shared so that others might understand the struggles, losses, fears, hopes, concerns, and grief of those concerned. They are shared to portray the uplifting moments too. These stories are not all sad and bad but much of what is revealed is not good.

Part I is concerned with bringing into the spotlight a problem in our communities that, hitherto, has not received sufficient attention. As you will have already seen, the Prologue introduced the problem of concern. Central to this was the lack of recognition of what these parents were dealing with and how little acknowledgement and support they received. A major objective of this work was to spotlight a neglected problem in our workplaces and communities; a source of work-home conflict not previously considered.

Chapter 1 canvasses several areas of literature of relevance to this study. First, the work-home conflict, specifically: issues such as the tension between mothering and working; the woman's 'ethic of care'; the different 'voice' of women; shifts in household working patterns, especially of women into the work force; and representations of 'home' and 'work' in organisations. Questions of gender and career are also considered, including some of the typical stumbling blocks facing women: discrimination (overt and covert); 'glass ceilings'; and the continuing struggle for women expected to work what Arlie Hochschild terms 'The Second Shift' (1989). The prevalence and increasing phenomenon of caregiving and working is also introduced. This is a significant problem, and one that touches families, communities and organisations worldwide. While the burden of caregiving still predominantly falls to women, many women are increasingly undertaking full-time paid work as well, whether through choice or need. The special challenges of caring for a child with chronic illness while working full-time are exposed.

Chapter 2 begins by introducing the nine women who participated in this study. The chapter continues to detail a unique action research journey. This action research project involved a unique utilisation of the philosophical orientations of Heideggerian phenomenology and naturalistic inquiry. The action research project included specific features that lent themselves exceedingly well to this study. There were two rounds of qualitative interviews conducted, each from a different perspective. In the first round, Stage 1, respondents were asked to share their experiences and feelings from a *retrospective* perspective; that is, what did you do? How did you feel about that? What happened? The second round of interviews, Stage 2, in contrast, asked respondents to think about their situation from a *prospective* perspective, that is: what would you do if you had your time over? What would you do (if anything) differently next time? What might change? Stage 2 also presented fictional vignettes to respondents for comment that were based largely on Stage 1 interview data. The vignettes focused on issues of particular interest such as: the availability of childcare; workplace disclosure and discrimination; career choices and sacrifices; and personal and work-related relationships. Third, respondents were invited to participate in a Culminating Group Experience which involved my sharing emergent themes, analysis and interpretations, via presentation, comment and discussion. Data from all three stages of the research was utilised to share these women's experiences. The chapters that follow include: extracted narratives from interviews; researcher reflections; and data poems (Moisiewicz, 2005). It is hoped that this combination of data offers a rich and rewarding depiction of these women's lives, made in an effort to improve their human condition.

Part II of the book moves to recognise and acknowledge the anguish of those who participated in this study. Chapter 3 introduces these women's experience of 'disconnection'; from colleagues, other mothers, and from partners, friends and family, with their sense of disconnectedness being largely related to their differing responsibilities, fears and concerns shouldered alongside their working lives. What repeatedly arose in the stories shared was these women's overwhelming sense of having to 'do it all'. It was always they who had to respond, take responsibility, plan, consider, and worry. Sadly, this combined to produce their definite sense that those around them rarely understood the continuing, multiple, conflicting and exhausting responsibilities they faced. Often, these women were alone in their caring responsibilities: where male partners were still present (and often, they were not), even in functional and supportive relationships, it was mostly the mother who received the call from the school (not their partner); it was she who took the child to the doctor, counseling, or the hospital, as was required. Sadly, however, in many cases, male partners were absent – physically, emotionally, or financially.

Chapter 4 acknowledges the grief these women experienced at work and at home as a result of their experiences. The chapter begins by talking about grief, and the need to acknowledge that 'there is always grief in the room', be it experienced by one who has lost a close family member, been diagnosed with a serious illness, or has lost their job. The grief these women experienced existed both at home and at work, and involved characteristics that are generally not included in traditional models of grief. As well as underscoring the grief and depression experienced, their ongoing, recurring and multiple sources of grief are underlined. Unlike a death in the family, their grief continued and was linked inexorably to the health and abilities of their child. Their fear and uncertainty for the future, especially as it related to their child, was something they carried with them everyday, at work and at home. As well as being ongoing, their grief had multiple sources: losses experienced by their child; shifts, changes and losses in their own lives; strained relationships; and lost income, career and leisure opportunities. Finally, the grief they experienced recurred: for these women, the chronic nature of their difficulties conspired such that daily events, large or small, acted as triggers. From the hospitalisation of their child to the thoughtless comment of a colleague; the grief they experienced was lived everyday – at home and at work – and needed to be acknowledged and understood.

Chapter 5 explores the cruelty and indifference that abounded in these women's social networks. The responses of the people around them – partners (and ex-partners), family members, friends, colleagues, health and educational professionals, and complete strangers – are shared. Unfortunately, much of what was shared involved episodes of callous thoughtlessness, even cruelty. Most surprising to me was the speed and frequency with which respondents were able to share recollections of cruel, thoughtless and insensitive incidents.

In Chapter 6, the theme of 'Clayton's Support'[1] is introduced and developed. Clayton's support is defined as the support you get when you are not getting support. These women shared example after example of promises and expectations of support from others that was far from the reality of the support received. This was a shocking revelation considering these women's unequivocal need for support in their lives. Their stories showed support being absent, uneven, hurtful and unhelpful, unreliable, diminishing and, importantly, widely disparate from was anticipated, wanted and needed.

Part III shifts the focus to enabling the survival of those who find themselves parenting a child with a chronic illness and working fulltime. Chapter 7 turns to the world of work, drawing attention to the problems and flawed assumptions that exist, and paying specific attention to the dilemmas and tensions surrounding working and caring, such as: the need to work; orientations towards flexible working conditions; inconstant support; ambivalence; disclosure issues; balancing working and caring; and work choices made. The social negotiations these women continually encountered, the adaptations and choices they made to enable them to continue working, including their concerns regarding their ability to progress in the workplace, are all considered. Examination of these issues depicts what might have helped these women and what might help others similarly placed in the future.

Chapter 8 concludes by returning to the research question posed, the substantive and methodological objectives set, confirming what has been achieved. Stories of survival, self, and work and home lives are included here with a focus on positive experiences. These are highlighted to offer a balanced view and so that others might learn positive approaches to gaining or giving support in the future. Chapter 8 concludes by returning to the need to move towards compassion and actionable knowledge as a means of working towards a brighter future.

Finally, this volume concludes with an Epilogue; a second and final fictional diary entry, offering an alternative to the Prologue 'day in the life' (Vallant, 2005) and based on what has been learned. This story presents, hopefully, a happier account. It is an opportunity for fiction to be used to encapsulate a landscape of potential reality. It is the only part of this book that is not based on, or reflective of, actual experiences, although it was developed based on what was learned along the way, standing as a goal to be sought. In this diary entry, carers are in abundance; support services are known about and affordable; a grandmother has greater sensitivity; a mother is more assertive in getting her needs met; medical help offers real alternatives; understanding and helpful work colleagues abound; and the life-world is awash with friends at the ready and a partner who shares the load. In this story, life is not bleak, overwhelming and without respite – but it is still challenging. I hope it will demonstrate how life can change, how the way forward might look, and how the future could be.

1
Caring and Working as Work-Home Conflict

Finding Carers

Partner is overseas
Mother available to pick up and drop
Fifteen dollars an hour to mind all day?
Huge – I just can't afford it.

A hundred and seventy a week for three afternoons
So, three of the five days covered –
Better than nothing
I'm grateful, but it's not cheap.

(Dolly, Interview 2: 3)

Dolly's words, captured in the data poem above, encapsulates the endless tussle that working parents have with finding carers to look after their child. The demands of caring for a child with chronic illness, combined with working full-time, are significant. Outcomes may include: unintended negative impacts on other children; conflicting career and home demands; loss of personal energy levels and lifestyle; increased stress and grief; insufficient support at work and at home; increased personal susceptibility to illness; and strained interpersonal relationships. While there have been studies about the important question of overlapping roles where workers also have family and caring responsibilities (eg, van Eyk, 1992; Van den Heuval, 1993a; 1993b; Wolcott, 1993; Sawyer and Spurrier, 1996; Eagle, Miles and Icenogle, 1997; Edwards and Rothbard, 1999; Erickson, Nichols and Ritter, 2000; Russell and Bowman, 2000), there have been no purely qualitative studies addressing the challenges faced by women caring for children with chronic illness, while also undertaking full-time work.

This chapter will explore issues of concern for working parents, especially working mothers, as they negotiate the challenges of working and caring. For the purposes of this research, a *child* is defined as a male or female person aged between birth and 18 years of age, based on the premise that up to 18 years spans the entire developmental period for a child. As a child matures, parental assistance requiring time away from work may still be required.[1] A *chronic illness* is defined as any *long-term health problem or disability* experienced by the child for at least six months (Vickers, Parris and Bailey, 2004; Vickers, 2005b; 2005c; 2005d; Vickers and Parris, 2005). This is a significant, ongoing illness or disability, requiring ongoing medical or professional intervention (via pharmacological or other treatment, visits to medical or other professional practitioners, or hospitalisation) to treat acute episodes and/or chronic problems associated with the illness or disability. This book focuses on the *challenges presented to the carer who is also working full-time*, rather than a medicalised definition of the child's condition (Vickers, Parris and Bailey, 2004; Vickers, 2005b; 2005c; Vickers and Parris, 2005). This is not a study about the child's experiences with illness or disability but, rather, the experiences and challenges presented to their parents as carers who also worked full-time (Vickers, Parris and Bailey, 2004; Vickers, 2005b; 2005c; Vickers and Parris, 2005). While both men and women were sought to participate in this study, only women participated (see Chapter 2). Necessarily, this demanded an unplanned – and very important – gender orientation for this work.

Several areas of literature are explored so that some of the wider questions pertaining to working motherhood and the work-life balance might be better understood, especially to frame the experiences and meanings shared in the chapters that follow. In this chapter, the discussion will assay the literature as follows:

- Children with chronic illness;
- The work-home conflict;
- Gender and work;
- Caring and working: an increasing phenomenon; and,
- The changing workplace.

Children with chronic illness

Flawed assumptions prevail – that children are predominantly healthy and unburdened by issues of illness and disability that commonly associate with age and infirmity. The vast majority still continue to believe that, should a health problem arise for a child, they will recover quickly as a result of the huge armamentarium of remedies available to the medical community that have long since halted the intrusion of chronic childhood disease and disability into our modern existence. However, children with chronic disease and illness are a significant group of the population (Martin and Nisa, 1996: 1). Newacheck (1994; cited in Melnyk et al, 2001) reported that approximately 31 per cent of children under the age of 18 years have one or more chronic illnesses (Vickers, Parris and Bailey, 2004; Vickers, 2005b; 2005c). While it is acknowledged that illness and disability tends to be associated with the ageing process, children are still at a significant risk of having a disability or long-term health condition due to accidents, environmental factors or through being born with a particular disorder (ABS, 2002: 5). Of the 3.9 million children in Australia aged 0–14 years in 1998, almost one in seven have a long-term health condition (594,600 or 15 per cent), with boys more likely (18 per cent) to be affected than girls (13 per cent). Paradoxically, as a result of the advances in scientific knowledge and technology, the number of children with a chronic illness is increasing (Gibson, 1995: 1201; Vickers, Parris and Bailey, 2004; Vickers, 2005b; 2005c).

Examples of children's medical diagnoses may include: cerebral palsy, muscular dystrophy, asthma, cystic fibrosis, diabetes, myelodysplasia, hydrocephalus, cleft palate, burns, cancer, or other physical disabilities as a result of trauma or congenital anomalies (Burke et al, 1999; Vickers, Parris and Bailey, 2004; Vickers, 2005b). As with adults, children with chronic illness are not necessarily faced with acute, life-threatening situations (although they may be); the central concern is the longer-term 'care' of the illness (Melnyk et al, 2001; O'Brien, 2001). Of particular interest are conditions that occur more frequently in this age group, such as asthma, attention deficit disorder/attention deficit and hyperactivity disorder (ADD/ADHD), intellectual and developmental disorders, and hearing or speech loss (ABS, 2002: 5).

Some conditions are especially problematic, providing numerous challenges. For example, asthma is the most common long-term health condition, affecting 312,000 children (8 per cent) aged 0–14 years (ABS, 2002: 5). As many as 21 per cent of males aged 5–14 years report having asthma, with females of the same age group reporting 17 per cent (ABS, 1999: 2). Working parents of a child with asthma know that asthma requires care, such as time to supervise medication use and to take affected children to the doctor. One of the primary tasks to interrupt a carer's work-life is the need to take children to the doctor (Van den Heuval, 1993b). While figures specific to *carers* of children with long-term health conditions were not available, one can intuitively see how these kinds of professional consultations would be difficult to repeatedly schedule for the full-time working parent. In Australia, for instance, one in four (25 per cent) of children aged less than five years had consulted a doctor in the previous two weeks; for children aged 5–14 years the proportion was 15 per cent (ABS, 2001: 7). These caring responsibilities flow into the workplace: for example, in 1995, the National Health Service (NHS) estimated that 1 in 26 children (or 3.8 per cent) aged 0–14 years with asthma had taken one or more days off school in the past two weeks because of their asthma (ABS, 1999: 3). Asthma causes disruption to the lives of children (ABS, 1999: 3) and, consequently, also to the working lives of their parents – usually their mothers. Just considering this single chronic illness, one can see how serious the issue of caregiving can be for workers, especially when considering all possible chronic conditions, multiple conditions that might exist, conditions requiring constant vigilance, or carers being responsible for other dependents.

For other conditions, the intrusion can also be significant and frequent. For example, ADD/ADHD is a condition increasingly being diagnosed, and one that can cause difficulties in learning. This would be troubling for parents concerned with their children's educational and employment possibilities in the future. Uncertainty and fear about the future is a constant worry for parents of children who are chronically ill (Melnyk et al, 2001; O'Brien, 2001). ADD/ADHD may also be responsible for behavioural problems; another serendipitous outcome that may also impact parental workers called away from work to respond. Nearly half (49 per cent) of children with ADD/ADHD have a profound or severe restriction on their lives, requiring some form of assistance (ABS, 2002: 5). For working parents, unscheduled time away from work would be a prevailing issue, as we will see.

Other concerns that relate to the child's diagnosis have been termed a chronic disaster (Erikson, 1994). After the difficulties associated with the diagnosis phase (Quittner et al, 1992), families have to then deal with the 'long haul' portion of the chronic phase (Rolland, 1987; Burke et al, 1999). The stressors encountered by parents of children with chronic illness are usually multiple and ongoing (Melnyk et al, 2001), and include stressors which vary over time, such as those experienced: (a) at the time of diagnosis; (b) during developmental transitions; (c) that are related to the ongoing healthcare needs of their child; and,

(d) that arise as their child experiences illness exacerbations and hospitalisations (Melnyk et al, 2001). Chronic illness presents different challenges at different life stages. For instance, early onset of chronic illness is interpreted differently by a small child, who may be concerned with abandonment or not understanding what is happening to them. Conversely, a child diagnosed during adolescence may be more concerned with what the future might hold, with bodily image, and the continuance of childlike dependency (Martin and Nisa, 1996: 3). These issues all affect families, and may involve parental intervention during the working week.

Parental responses to the diagnosis of their child's chronic condition commonly include shock, disbelief, denial, and anger – the traditional grief responses (Austin, 1990; Canam, 1993; Eakes, 1995; Melnyk et al, 2001). Other responses commonly reported include despair, depression, frustration and confusion (Eakes, 1995; Melnyk et al, 2001). In addition to this, feelings of guilt, decreased self-worth and a lack of confidence are also common (Stevens, 1994; Melnyk et al, 2001). The term chronic sorrow (Olshansky, 1962; Melnyk et al, 2001) describes a coping mechanism that allows for periodic grieving. It is thought to be a recurring phenomenon, rather than an ongoing, continuous process (Winkler, 1981; Melnyk et al, 2001). The grief experienced by the women in this study is explored more fully in Chapter 4.

Changes in the child's or family's status quo can also trigger stressors, sometimes unexpectedly; for example, a hospitalisation (Sawyer and Spurrier, 1996; Burke et al, 1999). Exacerbations are common with chronic illness. Deterioration in the child's health over time may also result in reduced functioning or quality of life, further taxing caregiving resources (Melnyk et al, 2001). Hospitalisations require parents to further divide their time between normal responsibilities and the hospitalised child (Melnyk et al, 2001) – even more difficult for those working full-time. Further, the varying and shifting nature of chronic illness can present problems, with families finding some issues less stressful at one point, that later become huge problems (Sawyer and Spurrier, 1996; Burke et al, 1999). A hospitalisation or other health event can also trigger unrelated family issues, as well as adding to the ongoing, unpredictable and hazardous nature of the illness (Burke et al, 1999).

Families often move locations because of the child's illness, for example, to be closer to medical assistance. Others may feel constrained to remain in a particular locale because of their dependence on care provision close at hand, or medical services required for their child. This can have a flow on effect to the caregiver's career; 42 per cent of families report some type of employment change because of the child's condition or necessary care (Burke et al, 1999). Such changes can result in less income, against the reality of expensive essentials associated with medical care. The financial burden of ongoing care may become a major stress for families. Not only is healthcare expensive, but the costs related to housing modifications, special equipment and other services can present additional financial demands on families (Melnyk et al, 2001), creating problems with other family expenses (Burke et al, 1999), and placing pressure on income providers.

Routine child rearing tasks can also become far more complex and challenging when a child has a chronic illness (Burke et al, 1999). For example, acute and recurrent distress frequently occurs as parents notice their child looking and responding differently from others, or delayed in development (Robson, 1997; Melnyk et al, 2001). It may be a crystallising moment for parents as they realise, for the first time, the extent to which the child is different from peers in physical or cognitive ability, or social skills (Melnyk et al, 2001). For example, the major step of a child entering the school system can become imbued with issues surrounding the need for the parent to give up control of the child's healthcare management during the day to teachers – who, unfortunately, may have little knowledge about childhood chronic illness (Melnyk et al, 2001). Parents still have to pay attention to work roles, often during stressful periods, with colleagues not understanding their experiences.

Similarly, day-to-day care for conditions such as cystic fibrosis (CF) can be time-consuming and stressful, on a regular basis (Quittner et al, 1992). Daily healthcare regimens are time-consuming, rigorous, unrelenting – taxing to both children and parents. Parents report that seeing their child in physical or emotional pain and discomfort is heart-wrenching and frequently triggers overwhelming feelings of guilt and inadequacy (Quittner et al, 1992; Simon and Smith, 1992; Melnyk et al, 2001). For some, taking a child to physical therapy may also be a tremendous burden; for others, it is regarded as positive progress toward enhancing their child's outcomes (Melnyk et al, 2001). Either way, holding down a full-time job adds immeasurably to the strain. Balancing the competing demands of care regimes, working and family responsibilities can be challenging and exhausting (Melnyk et al, 2001). The impact of chronic disease on children and families is less related to the actual diagnosis than to the illness and disability profile and its impact on family functioning (Martin and Nisa, 1996; Sawyer and Spurrier, 1996). The diagnosis of a chronic condition of any child places the physical health and emotional well-being of all the members of that family at risk (Martin and Nisa, 1996: 3). I now move the discussion into the realm of the work-home conflict. This is a growing problem as women's participation in the labour force continues to grow, and women continue to shoulder most of the responsibility for home duties.

The work-home conflict

'Social settlement' in Australia described post-World War II family roles in terms of the male breadwinner and female carer of the household. Men and women had very traditional roles, and were mostly married. At that time, men numerically dominated the workforce (Hancock, 2002: 121) and middle class women were assumed to be fit for one job only, that of a housewife (Gutek, 2001: 379). However, the assumptions underpinning this post-war way of life are fast dissolving, especially over the past two decades. One area of change has been the increasing diversification of employment relationships with regards to tenure, hours and location (Hancock, 2002: 122). Work can be, potentially, a great positive for individuals, families and societies. It can be a source of pride, fulfilment and social networks, offering structure to lives while enabling food, shelter, personal care, and other goods and services necessary for a high quality life (Gjerdingen et al, 2000: 2). Work plays a prominent role in women's lives, increasingly so, as more women have assumed responsibility for paid employment in addition to family and household tasks (Gjerdingen et al, 2000: 2). Work is important; a major part of our lives is occupied in work and work-related activities. Job and life satisfaction are closely related (Jena, 1999: 75).

However, women continue to take primary responsibility for the care of children and for associated domestic work (Giordano, 1995: 5). The traditional division of labour between men and women in the home has shown remarkable resilience, even alongside dramatic changes in women's participation in the paid workforce (Baxter, 2000: 12). For most women, adding the role of paid worker to their lives has not resulted in the removal of marital and parental responsibilities (Giordano, 1995: 5). Women undertaking paid work find themselves working two shifts: one for their employer and one in the home (Hochschild, 1989). Unfortunately, the rise in numbers of women who have entered paid employment since the end of World War II has not seen a comparable rise in men's levels of participation in unpaid work in the home (Baxter, 2000: 12).[2] The result remains that women continue to juggle multiple responsibilities in various settings, including households, workplaces and communities (Giordano, 1995: 5; Gjerdingen et al, 2000: 3). Women still retain primary responsibility for providing or finding childcare, and taking care of domestic chores (Albelda and Tilly, 1998: 43). Even high achieving women who are married continue to carry the lion's share of domestic responsibilities (Hewlett, 2002: 70).

These kinds of structural shifts in labour patterns (among others) have created the work-home conflict. Much research has been undertaken into the work-home conflict (see, for example, Greenhaus and Beutell, 1985; Hochschild, 1989; Hopfl, 1992; Van den Heuval, 1993a; Schein, 1993; Hochschild, 1997; Kinnunen and Mauno, 1998; Clark, 2000; Gjerdingen et al, 2000; Clark, 2001; Casper et al, 2002; Cinamon and Rich, 2002; Vickers, 2001b; Vickers and Parris, 2005). Labour force participation of women has risen dramatically in the last century (Gjerdingen et al, 2000; Kurz, 2000). The working woman is not a variation from the norm; she is now considered to be the norm (Giordano, 1995: 4). This increased involvement of women in the workforce has been called the 'subtle revolution' (Smith, 1979; cited in Sharpe, Hermsen and Billings, 2002: 78) because it forced a rethinking of societal norms regarding the division of work and family responsibilities, and the role of employers in assisting employees meet their family-related demands (Sharpe, Hermsen and Billings, 2002: 78). However, the 'revolution' has had limited impact. Gender stereotypes remain not only descriptive, but prescriptive, especially for women. They denote not only differences in how women and men actually are, but also dictate norms of how they *should* be (Terborg, 1977; Eagly, 1987; Burgess and Borgida, 1999; Heilman, 2001: 659).

Discussion of the work-family conflict has focused on, among other things, the strain that can develop when balancing the demands of work and family (Greenhaus and Beutell, 1985). For many women today, a high level of conflict and increased time pressures are experienced as they deal with substantial family responsibilities and significant workloads (Casper et al, 2002; Cinamon and Rich, 2002). Several unique stressors have been identified which employed women encounter at work: the marriage-work interface; social isolation; discrimination; and stereotyping (Jena, 1999: 76). In addition to these employment issues, family and households are also sources of continuous work, particularly when children are present in the home. On average, women invest considerably more time in the work of family and household than do men, an observation made in both national and international studies (Gjerdingen et al, 2000: 5). In fact, women's work within the home is often reported to be *double or more* than that of men's, a pattern confirmed in the United States, Sweden and the Netherlands (Gjerdingen et al, 2000: 5; emphasis added). The impact of having a young child on housework is also noted as being greater for the wife than for the husband (Kiker and Ng, 1990; Gjerdingen et al, 2000: 7). As we will see (especially in Chapter 3), this asymmetry of responsibility is even more stark when women have a child with a chronic illness.

New working patterns, including the expansion of long working hours (Perrons, 2003: 68), have contributed to the problem by eroding the usual boundaries and rhythms of working life, with the concept and reality of a fixed working day declining (Perrons, 2003: 69). The shift from the 'neo-traditional' strategy of middle class – the traditional breadwinner-homemaker model – shows men working considerably longer hours (Moen and Elliot, 2003: 591). However, women are now also working longer paid hours too. And what happens to working women who also have to care for a child with a chronic illness? What happens if there is no husband, or he doesn't work at all? Even for the women who participated in this study who reported supportive partners (just one-third), the time bind experienced and the imbalance of responsibilities during their 'second shift' was evident (Vickers and Parris, 2005). Studies continue to show that women from dual career households not only continue to do a larger share of the housework and childcare, but continue to carry the *primary* responsibility for these tasks (Gjerdingen et al, 2000: 7).

The continuing struggle with managing 'The Second Shift' (Hochschild, 1989) and 'The Time Bind' (Hochschild, 1997) is worth our attention, especially in light of the likelihood of these women's additional home responsibilities. The time bind experienced by working women and men dealing with the dual responsibilities of home and work (Hochschild 1997; Roxburgh, 2002) remains unresolved. For parents who are also carers of a child with chronic illness, it remains relatively untouched. The consideration of the multiple roles of women – at home and at work – and the demands of each role in terms of time, energy and commitment (Kinnunen and Mauno, 1998) is essential. There are a tremendous number of work-related difficulties with which women are expected to cope (Giordano, 1995: 4). One of these is the sheer volume of work that women are expected to do. A national longitudinal study conducted in the United States showed that the total workload for employed women of all ages was nearly 4000 hours per year, compared to 3400 hours for men. This translates into an average of 80 hours of work per week (paid and unpaid) for women, compared to just 68 hours for men (Gjerdingen et al, 2000: 7). The problem is compounded as women are continually reminded that they can, and should, 'have it all' (Hewlett, 2002: 70) – they wanted choices in love, life and work that men take for granted, including a purpose beyond themselves to help them cope with their own mortality (Hewlett, 2002: 70). However, the flawed belief that women can have it all is one that secures much guilt, stress and self-doubt for those seeking it.

Hewlett (2002: 68) highlights the 'time crunch' for women, especially in relation to dealing with long and lengthening workweeks. Hancock (2002: 119) speaks of the 'care crunch', where changing work landscapes, family structures and welfare offerings are impacting on the capacity of households and families to cope. In addition to acknowledging the volume of additional hours women work, debate has also now arisen as to whether occupying these multiple roles (eg, wife, mother, carer, worker) is beneficial or detrimental to one's well-being. While there is note of the 'healthy worker effect', where those who work are more likely to be healthier than those who do not (Gjerdingen et al, 2000: 8), the opposing concept, role strain, purports that some role combinations can be detrimental to one's well-being due to competing demands on one's time, energy and involvement. There is now evidence that certain characteristics of work roles, either separately or in combination, may contribute to physical, mental, or marital problems (Gjerdingen et al, 2000: 9) – something we will see explicitly in the chapters that follow. There is certainly evidence that these multiple roles can impact negatively on physical and mental health, and marital well-being (Gjerdingen et al, 2000). For instance, women with three or more children report poorer physical health, and just being a parent is associated with headaches, exhaustion, overeating, smoking and drinking (Langan-Fox and Poole, 1995: 113). The stresses of parenting, caring and working are real.

Then consider, in combination with the above, the strain associated with occupational stress (Langan-Fox and Poole, 1995; Jena, 1999): the imbalance resulting from job-related demands and abilities. Occupational stress involves two main areas: sources of stress at work and individual characteristics (Langan-Fox and Poole, 1995: 113). However, it is also recognised as a far more complex phenomenon that develops through the interaction of the person-environment process (Lazarus and Launier, 1978; Mitchell et al, 1988; Langan-Fox and Poole, 1995: 114). There is considerable evidence that psychological and social stressors do have negative effects on the physical and mental health of the worker, and employed women experience greater stress than both unemployed women and employed men (Jena, 1999: 75). Gender differences show that women experience stressful life events in terms of psychological stress, such as anxiety and emotional disturbances (Jena, 1999: 76). Once again, while a certain amount of stress can be beneficial to health and act as a catalyst for optimum performance, too much stress has long been recognised as being damaging to one's health and well-being (Langan-Fox and Poole, 1995: 113). Occupational stress can exact a heavy toll on employees in terms of mental and physical health and a much reduced quality of life. It is also expensive to employers (Langan-Fox and Poole, 1995: 113), and harmful to individuals and families.

Gender and work

For women, work lives and work learning are woven into family and other relations with fluidity and complexity, and are marked by struggles critical to their sense of self (Fenwick, 1998: 199). The increased presence of women in the workplace and their assumption of new roles, unfortunately, does not appear to preclude gender-stereotypic perceptions (Heilman, 2001: 658). Traditional stereotypes continue to predominate at work and at home (Heilman, 2001: 658). Many of the typical and well-acknowledged career blocks for women still exist: gender stereotypes; discrimination; 'glass ceilings'; the 'mommy track'; inequitable pay; the pervasiveness of male values and organisational cultures; interrupted career paths; as well as women's continued over-representation in part-time, lower paid and lower status work. These issues need to be considered, especially in light of the needs of women also caring for a child with chronic illness.

Gender equality within the paid labour market has been an important goal of second wave feminism (Baxter, 2000: 14). Not only have feminists recognised the importance of equal wages and equal access to employment as being fundamental to women's fight for independence from men, but the 'right to work' is seen as a central component of modern citizenship (Baxter, 2000: 14). Unfortunately, not only have feminists not always been united in their efforts to achieve gender equality at work, but clearly other organisational, community and social impediments continue to stand in the way, not the least of which is the expectation that women retain primary responsibility for family well-being, even if this comes at their expense.

Until relatively recently, for example, the term 'managerial careers' still referred only to men and *their* traditional career which was one that involved an uninterrupted climb (with varying degrees of success) up a hierarchical ladder (Schneer and Reitman, 1995: 290). Unfortunately, women continue to experience several basic sources of workplace impediments: role choice or role overload; sex-based and other wage discrimination; occupational sex segregation; and the underutilisation of their abilities (Giordano, 1995: 5). Despite discriminatory expectations and assumptions to the contrary, women can and do contribute effectively to our workplaces – when they are allowed to – even when they have a child with a chronic illness. However, the constant interference of family and caregiving responsibilities can hinder women's career progression, decrease satisfaction with work, interfere with concentration on the job, as well as increase absenteeism and possibly employee turnover (Wentling, 1998: 18; Vickers and Wilkes, 2004). These are issues that should be of concern to individuals, families, communities and workplaces.

Women's careers tend to be characterised, more than men's, by periods of interruption and alternative work arrangements. Many women also work part-time (Bierema, 1998: 96) which can have a very negative impact on careers and financial standing, especially over the longer-term. Women also tend to still work predominantly in gender-specific areas that align comfortably with gender stereotypical expectations of how women 'should be'. Gender stereotypes tend to represent and relate to attributes that are highly valued for each sex. For women, traits that are positively valued and are central to their 'shoulds' tend to be the nurturing and communal traits (Heilman, 2001: 659). Women, thus, are frequently still encouraged to take up traditional care-related roles: nursing, teaching, and administrative support roles, which are traditionally paid much less than male-dominated professions such as medicine, engineering, and business management. That said, in the past 20 years, the proportions of women in medicine, law, clinical psychology, management and accounting have increased much more rapidly than they have in other areas (Gutek, 2001: 380). However, while women are the fastest growing segment of the labour force, they are still disproportionately employed in slow-growing or declining occupations (Giordano, 1995: 5). Breaking from the stereotypical mold, as the women in this study often did, is quite an achievement.

Women also tend to be still segregated into typically female careers that perpetuate the traditional, gender-specific wage gap that accompanies this (Bierema, 1998: 96). When women choose a career that breaks with tradition, they bring qualities that are not necessarily valued in that career, and do not always know the 'rules' for success. Due to continuing gender stereotypes, women can expect to be on slower tracks than men as they are expected to be less committed to their careers due to their family obligations (Schneer and Reitman, 1995: 291). They can also expect to earn less. In the US, women's earnings are considerably lower than men's – approximately 70 cents to every man's dollar.

Gender stereotypes have been demonstrated, over and over, to have a deleterious effect on women's career progression. The 'glass ceiling' (Snyder, 1993; Albelda and Tilly, 1998: 43; Heilman, 2001: 657) – defined by the US Department of Labor (1991) as a composite of artificial barriers based on attitudinal or organisational bias that prevent qualified [women] from advancing upward in their organisation into [senior] management level positions – is as impenetrable as ever (Snyder, 1993). This barrier will be felt at some point in a woman's career, and is somehow viewed as a natural consequence of gender stereotypes (Heilman, 2001: 657). Women, especially those with children, will ultimately hit the glass ceiling – that invisible barrier to further advancement – and are subsequently shunted off to the 'mommy track' (Snyder, 1993: 100; Albelda and Tilly, 1998: 43). Others, particularly single mothers with limited skills or support, are stuck in the bottomless pit of poverty (Albelda and Tilly, 1998: 43). Being competent provides no assurance that a woman will advance to the same organisational levels as an equivalently performing male (Heilman, 2001: 657). When one adds the need to undertake the vast majority of household tasks, and the responsibility of caring for a child with chronic illness, we see women so placed at an extreme disadvantage.

It is recognised that different communication styles between men and women affect the way they perceive each other and the way they work together (Zanetic and Jeffery, 1995: 13). Male managers have assumed – automatically – that women with children are not interested in promotions or important developmental assignments requiring longer hours (Snyder, 1993: 100). However, while the suggestion that the first step towards change in organisations might be to recognise that different communication styles exist (Zanetic and Jeffery, 1995:

13), it is still the case that patriarchal segregation and systemic discrimination still plague female workers, with systemic discrimination being especially prevalent in work systems designed and controlled by white males (Bierema, 1998: 97; Giordano, 1995: 5). Women in the work force find themselves having to adapt to organisations based on male values, attitudes, history and culture (Zanetic and Jeffery, 1995: 13). Those male values and attitudes rarely leave room for empathic support for one whose workday is interrupted because of a sick child.

Caring and working: an increasing phenomenon

The worldwide prevalence and increasing phenomenon of informal care provision is a significant and growing problem, and one that touches families, communities and organisations worldwide, as populations continue to age and governments struggle to find ways to provide for those in need. One path many governments have chosen is to push the provision of care back to communities and away from the more traditional, formal care provision that has previously been available in many parts of the world. This shift to informal care provision by families and communities (Vickers and Parris, 2005) can result in the further fragmentation of community care services that have long been recognised as problematic in Australia, although the problem is by no means confined to Australia (Fine, 1999: 68). With a health and welfare system increasingly emphasising outcomes and cost effectiveness, the co-ordination of services between hospitals, residential care, community care services and other healthcare providers has become imperative (Fine, 1999). Attempts by governments of different political persuasions across the English-speaking world to reduce expenditure have been a major factor in the search for improved co-ordination. The attempts that have been made seem all the more urgent by difficulties that consumers experience gaining access to services and the apparent failure of some government programmes to accomplish their aims (Fine, 1999: 70).

As noted earlier, women still primarily tackle the role of caregiving for children (Robinson and Godbey, 1999; Mattingly and Bianchi, 2003). However, shifts from institutionalised care to informal care provision in both eldercare and care for people with disabilities, together with established and seemingly immutable roles for women as primary care providers for dependent children, creates more strain and responsibility for women, as do increased female paid work participation rates all over the Western world (Vickers and Parris, 2005). Such caring responsibilities entail the physical demands of care as well as the 'mental work' of worry, seeking advice and finding information (Renzetti and Curran, 1999: 166).

In Australia, 70 per cent of primary caregivers are female, with 70 per cent of these caregivers caring for a person in the same household (ABS, 1998: 10). Recent estimates indicate that over half of all women will provide care for someone who is ill or disabled at some point in their life (Pavalko and Artis, 1997: 170). In the age group 35–44 years, approximately 75 per cent of primary carers were women, as against just 22 per cent of men (ABS, 1998: 10). In the age group 45–54 years, women undertaking primary caregiving was as high as 79 per cent, with males well below 40 per cent (ABS, 1998: 10). Women continue to be the main providers of informal eldercare around the world (Jutras and Veilleux, 1991: 2; Farkas and Himes, 1997: 180; Pavalko and Artis, 1997: 170; Doty, Jackson and Crown, 1998: 335; Lee, 2001), not just in Australia, providing another significant barrier for career paths.

Of interest, an estimated 307,500 (15 per cent) of all carers were self-employed. Of these, 49,200 (16 per cent) started their own business, or became a contractor, because it made it easier for them to provide care. Once again, women were more likely than men to do this because it made caring responsibilities easier (29 per cent compared to 9 per cent) (ABS, 2000: 2). Finally, an estimated 573,900 (29 per cent) of all carers were *not* looking for paid work. Of these, 228,000 (40 per cent) were not looking for work primarily *because* of their caring responsibilities. Once again, this was higher for females (47 per cent) than males (12 per cent) (ABS, 2000: 30), demonstrating the prevailing expectations that women sacrifice their work and remain as primary caregivers (ABS, 2000).

Living with chronic conditions can be very difficult for both the child involved, and for their parents and siblings (Martin and Nisa, 1996). The problem is 'invisible' and potentially traumatising. Concern for children whose mothers work has been neglected for many years (Kurz, 2000: 435). Women have traditionally been socialised to an 'ethic of care' (Stohs, 1994; Doty, Jackson and Crown, 1998: 332), feeling compelled to be attentive and responsive to the needs of individual family members (Doty, Jackson and Crown, 1998: 332). Indeed, women have been socialised to value highly the maintenance of supportive relationships at the expense of their own health or economic position (Vickers and Parris, 2005). The ethic of care encourages women – at any age – to voluntarily make choices that can be detrimental to their physical, personal and economic well-being (Lee, 2001:

395). While the provision of care may provide emotional satisfaction, it does come at a personal cost (Lee, 2001: 394). It is still the case that women are assumed to be the 'natural' ones to provide care for others (Rasmussen, 2004); caring is viewed as a natural talent of women (Jenkins, 2004) and women are assumed to be the ones to have the necessary caring credentials (Jenkins, 2004). However, even the majority of research in this area fails to challenge the disproportionate number of women providing care, with researchers often making the same assumptions made by broader society and by caregivers themselves (Vickers and Parris, 2005) – that it is somehow natural and inevitable that women will take up the burden of care, without payment or recognition (Lee, 2001: 394; Vickers and Wilkes, 2004); that it is 'her job' (Vickers, Parris and Bailey, 2004).

For many women undertaking full-time paid work, not only are they still responsible for the majority of household tasks and responsibilities, childcare, homemaking and relationship nurturance, they are now also expected to contribute financially to the household in a significant way (Vickers and Wilkes, 2004). As informal care provision increasingly moves onto the agenda for this generation, additional caring responsibilities will provide one more thing for women to add to their already disturbingly long list of responsibilities and roles (Vickers and Wilkes, 2004). Gendered expectations (Rasmussen, 2004) continue to find women being expected to take up care-related activities for family members and relatives, regardless of the economic, personal and emotional cost to themselves (Vickers and Parris, 2005). Not only are workplaces 'greedy' in their demands of workers, families are greedy too (Rasmussen, 2004). Gender stereotypes of women and men continue to predominate in both work and nonwork settings (Heilman, 2001: 658). When those caring responsibilities include a child with a significant chronic illness, the 'second shift' (Hochschild, 1989; Hewlett, 2002: 70) for women becomes a grave cause for concern.

The changing workplace

Trends in labour force participation rates have prompted changes in work arrangements. Many employers have implemented family-friendly workplace policies designed to help harried workers meet conflicting work and family responsibilities (Baxter, 2000: 13; Sharpe, Hermsen and Billings, 2002: 79). Employers are offering employees various work options that were not possible under previous, more traditional, work arrangements. 'Family responsive' workplace polices include: reduced work hours to provide more time for family responsibilities; flexibility in scheduling work hours, with no reduction in the number of work hours; and provision of other resources, such as childcare or eldercare facilities (Sharpe, Hermsen and Billings, 2002: 80). Other workplace policies introduced in Australia include parental leave and flexibility in work hours (Baxter, 2000: 13). The availability of leave and flexible work arrangements, as well as a favourable attitude toward those entitlements on the part of employers and coworkers, are important issues for many (Baxter, 2000: 13). However, policies are of little help if coworkers and management are not supportive of their implementation.

Caring responsibilities can be very difficult, with both physical and emotional strain an outcome (Jenkins, 2004). A US study found that 40 to 50 per cent of employed women experience conflict, guilt and stress about their dual roles (Wentling, 1998: 17). While it is recognised that flexible work practices and policies may ease this burden, as long as organisations continue to reward the full commitment of employees, utilising flexible arrangements can be a liability for the careers of women (Wentling, 1998: 20). Indeed, such policies are still considered to be 'her' family policies; so much so that flexible working arrangements have been declared the defeat of mothers struggling to humanise the workplace. The evidence of defeat is seen in traditional workplace structures still not giving precedence to women's interests, needs, and identities as they continue as the exhausted worker bees of society (Moriarty, 2000: 55; Vickers and Parris, 2005). Flexible work polices may formally exist, but many workplaces are informally operating in a manner that do not support their use.

Unfortunately, the need for flexibility can push women to rely on multiple part-time roles, at great potential detriment to them financially over the long-term. The increased casualisation of the workforce in Australia and across the Western world, brings with it fewer benefits, rights and entitlements, creating situations where casual workers can find themselves vulnerable to low pay and multiple forms of employment insecurity in terms of such things as job tenure, work hours and representation (Hancock, 2002: 122). Casual employees, defined by the Australian Bureau of Statistics (ABS) as employees not entitled to either annual or sick leave in their main job, almost tripled between 1982 and 1999, from 700,000 to almost 2 million workers. The proportion of casual workers over the same period increased from 13.3 per cent to 26.4 per cent (Campbell, 2000; Hancock, 2002: 123).

Finally, I spotlight another issue of concern in contemporary workplaces: workplaces being hostile and abusive. This is not a new concept and has been closely linked with managerialist and capitalist doctrines. However, I raise this as a spectre for those who also have responsibilities and challenges outside of work. The concept of organisations being unreasonable and hurtful places is not new. Both Fromm (1942/1960; 1963/1994) and Blauner (1964) described organisations as alienating places, discussing feelings of fragmentation, meaninglessness, isolation and powerlessness in the capitalist workplace. Braverman (1994) discussed the degradation of work, while Marx (1975/1994) described the alienated workforce. All of these outcomes can be magnified when a staff member is also dealing with personal problems outside the workplace, especially if they feel unsupported or even under attack.

Powell (1998: 95) described an abusive workplace as a workplace that 'operates with callous disregard for its employees, not even displaying what might be considered a minimum amount of concern for their human needs'. Bullying, abuse and aggression in organisations is also being increasingly recognised as extremely harmful, and may be exacerbated by economic pressures and globalising economies. It may also be exacerbated for individuals already under enormous strain. Bullies often target vulnerable people, knowingly making use of organisational change processes to abuse their targets (Hutchinson et al, 2005a; 2005b). The literature on workplace aggression (Neuman and Baron, 1997; Felson, 2000), bullying in the workplace (Randall, 1997; Vickers, 2001c; Hutchinson et al, 2005a; 2005c), and workplace psychological abuse (Mann, 1996; Vickers, 2004) is increasing in its prevalence, with attention being increasingly turned to workplace-related physical, emotional and psychological abuse. Bullying and associated psychological, emotional, physical and verbal abuse, has been linked quite convincingly to torture (Mann, 1996; Vickers, 2001c). Further, structural changes and downsizing increasingly emphasise the managerialist emphasis in organisational life, making it increasingly difficult for parents to balance work and family so as to spend time with their children (Bianchi, 2000), especially if management have little personal sympathy for their plight or are using organisational change processes to make life more difficult (Hutchinson et al, 2005a; 2005b). More intensive emphasis on nondisease dimensions of chronic illness is required to improve life outcomes, especially for families (Martin and Nisa, 1996).

I turn now to Chapter 2, to introduce the respondents in this study and to describe the important methodological issues that proved central to this research. Readers less concerned with methodological choices might be encouraged, after meeting the respondents, to move directly to Part II of this book, to Chapters 3, 4, 5 and 6 (in whichever order you choose) which may be read independently, to learn about these women's lives. However, for those interested in methodology, Chapter 2 articulates the interesting and innovative research choices made. Enjoy.

2
A Useful Research Design

Remembering

I still remember getting teary and upset
I thought I'd resolved a lot
But still things cut deep to the bone
Sometimes, you do feel guilty.
It's not unreasonable to want to work
Kevin is a big part of my life, not my whole life.

I'm glad I participated
I looked forward to this
I enjoyed talking about Kevin
A chance to reflect, to think
You realise you're not alone
It's wonderful to get that.

(Evalyn, Interview 2: 19; CGE: 1)

This chapter details a unique research design. The action research orientation and actionable knowledge outcomes that arose from this research methodology, design and process were quite distinctive and allowed the research to proceed with respondents feeling like participants in a process, rather than objects of a study. The main objective, to improve the human condition (action research exists to promote liberating social change), involved learning and engagement by both researcher and respondent. I used a multi-method design, including the philosophical perspectives of Heideggerian phenomenology and naturalistic inquiry (Vickers, 2005e).

As signposts for the reader, the sections in this chapter will include the following:

- Introducing the participants;
- The research question;
- Action research to improve the human condition;
- An insider-outsider perspective;
- A unique research design; and,
- Doing the research: how it worked.

In this chapter, I have elected to include data, not to demonstrate substantive themes per se, but to depict the developmental process of the project, and how various stages succeeded in capturing relevant and meaningful data. Also depicted is a project being influenced by researcher choice, and respondents' being influenced by research. Sandelowski (1994: 46) tells us that scholarship can at once be rigorous and imaginative, interesting and beautifully rendered. I have tried to create a research report that is readable, informative and artful. I have deliberately avoided, as Sandelowski would have, depicting these women's lives in a pseudo-scientific manner. I saw my job as delivering these women's stories, meanings and experiences as accurately as I could, while enticing readers. I begin by introducing these marvellous women.

Introducing the participants

All respondents and their family members are identified with a pseudonym to protect their confidentiality. I introduce them to provide contextual information about their lives. Details are shared as they were relayed at the time of interview. On occasion, some contextual details have been modified very slightly to further protect the privacy of respondents and their children.

Dolly was a partner in a Human Resources (HR) consulting firm. She reported a significant career in senior HR management and policy development in large corporations. Dolly's daughter, Maggie (then four years old), started having major seizures – up to 20 per day and 20 minutes long – at about four months of age, after receiving a routine immunisation injection. Maggie's seizures resulted in her subsequent intellectual disability. Dolly had recently separated from her marital partner, Steven, who moved in with his girlfriend of many years just around the corner from where Dolly lived. Steven was Dolly's professional partner in their HR consulting firm.

Wendy was a head teacher at a Technical and Further Education (TAFE) College with many years experience in the education sector. At the time of interview, Wendy had just learned that her 16-year-old daughter, Samantha, had a form of muscular dystrophy, a multi-systemic, progressive and hereditary condition, passed on to Samantha by her father and Wendy's former partner. This condition promised wide-ranging outcomes including intellectual disability, wheelchair use, and general muscular deterioration. Samantha was struggling to complete her final year in high school.

Evalyn held a senior financial management position in a large public sector organisation. She was married to Ivan, a pharmacist, who owned his own business. Evalyn had two sons: Kevin and Mathew. Kevin had severe epilepsy with his numerous seizures ultimately also resulting in brain damage and significant intellectual disability. Kevin was nine years old. Evalyn reported a very supportive partnership with her husband, although she acknowledged towards the end of the project, that the ultimate weight of responsibility for planning and responding to Kevin's needs remained primarily with her. Evalyn's greatest fear was wondering who would care for her son when she could not.

Cate worked in the disability services industry. Cate's son, William, then four years old, had autism, diagnosed when he was just two. She cared for and financially supported two dependent children, a brother with a disability, and her husband. When Cate was growing up, her father had also become disabled. Cate shared that her husband, Colin, was not very supportive, and drank a great deal. She had never spoken to her husband about their child's disability and feared, deep down, that he blamed her. Cate had overheard Colin tell members of his own immediate family how 'disappointed' he was with their son.

Charlene's son, Jamie, was paraplegic as a result of his father (now separated from Charlene) having run over him. Jamie had also had to deal with serious bouts of pneumonia, at least twice a year, which Charlene still found terribly distressing to talk about. Charlene had worked three part-time jobs to support herself and her son. She also reported being taken to court by her ex-partner, who tried to sue her for being an unfit mother. She won the case – but had to find the time and money for the court battle around everything else.

Sandra's son, Edward, had Attention Deficit Disorder (ADD). In addition to this, he had chronic tonsillitis as a baby, up until the age of two, necessitating Sandra keeping him with her at all times (even while working). Edward had changed schools many times as a result of ADD-related difficulties with concentration, behaviour and anger-management. Sandra reported one incident when Edward threatened Sandra, and his sister Katrina, with a knife during an angry rage. Sandra worried that Edward was depressed and that, ultimately, he might commit suicide because of the loss and despair ADD was bringing to his life. Sandra was the managing director of a large, successful, HR recruitment agency. Sandra reported that her husband, Robert, had remained emotionally distant from Edward's problems and from Sandra over many years.

Oitk (One-Income-Two-Kids) had a daughter, Belinda, with scleroderma, a very rare autoimmune disease resulting in disintegration of the tissue in her leg. As a result, Belinda had a withered right leg, and was shortly to undergo a gruesome treatment, involving a wire cage being screwed – through the bone – to lengthen Belinda's leg. Belinda had an identical twin sister, Susan, who had recently been acting out and deliberately seeking attention from her mother. Oitk, a single mother, worked as a receptionist and was studying psychology at university.

Polly's son, Thomas, was born with Down's syndrome. Thomas was seven years old at the time of interview and had also been diagnosed, at the age of four, with leukaemia. Fortunately, at the time of interview, Thomas' leukaemia was in remission. Polly had worked in numerous very highly paid senior executive positions in large corporations in previous years, although, in recent times, she had chosen to pursue her career in the public sector because of the flexible hours and diminished responsibilities. Polly also lived with her daughter, Christine, and her husband, Clive, a very high profile author.

Sally's daughter, Nadine, now 16, was born with hydrocephalus (fluid in the brain), lipoma (a benign tumour in her brain), a midline cleft to the face, and no corpus callosum (the broad band of nervous tissue that connects the left and right hemispheres of the brain). Sally was a senior nursing manager responsible for the emergency department in a large Sydney metropolitan hospital. Sally's partner, Peter, was also a nurse, and she had two sons, Adam and Jeffrey. Sally reported that her husband, Peter, while very easy-going and supportive in some respects, had let her take the load for caring, planning and being responsible for Nadine's care over the years, especially when this involved tussles with the medical profession.

The research question

All good research starts with the identification of a problem (Erlandson et al, 1993). The research question for this project, you will recall (from Chapter 1) was:

What is life like for a full time worker who also cares for a child with a chronic illness?

When considering methodological questions, the question is not about *which* methodology is better than another, nor the respective merits or deficiencies of each. It is, rather, about selecting the methodology that is most suitable for the project (Sarantakos, 1993: 106). This research project was exploratory. Exploratory studies are carried out when there is insufficient information about the topic, making the formulation of a suitable hypothesis and the subsequent operationalisation of the research question difficult (Sarantakos, 1993: 114; Vickers, 2001a: 30). There was no current theory to test in this case, ruling out the use of more quantitative methods (Sarantakos, 1993: 15; Vickers, 2001a: 30). This project was undertaken to find out if it was feasible or necessary to carry out a larger one. It was also designed to uncover and generate new ideas, views and opinions, and to bring an under-researched area into the spotlight for debate (Vickers, 2001a: 30). While there has been considerable research about the experience of people caring for children with chronic illness and disability (eg Rolland, 1987; Austin, 1990; Simon and Smith, 1992; Canam, 1993; Stevens, 1994; Eakes, 1995; Martin and Nisa, 1996: 3; Robson, 1997; Burke et al, 1999; Melnyk et al, 2001), there was insufficient research into the perspective of people who also worked full-time.

Action research to improve the human condition

It has been suggested that social scientists carry a special burden of responsibility. It is necessary but not enough that the profession engage in disinterested pursuit of knowledge. It must encourage and support within itself scientific work that has as its aim the mutual enrichment of social sciences and the practical affairs of man [*sic*]. (Emery, 1977: 206)

The methodological choices for this action research project show how the evolving nature of the project contributed significantly to what action research ultimately seeks to do – to improve the human condition (Vickers, 2005e). Action research exists to promote liberating social change (Greenwood, 2002: 128; Vickers, 2005e). As with Emery and Thorsrud's (1975: 1) study, the first stage of this project concentrated on the experiences of participants, while the latter stages moved towards opportunities for human development and social change

(Vickers, 2005e). Like Emery (1977: 1), I was seeking ways in which examining and changing the conditions for participants could assist in making their future. This project focused on the lives of people who worked full-time while also caring for a child with a chronic illness.[1] Balancing these competing demands, while maintaining personal and family responsibilities, was likely to be challenging and exhausting (Melnyk et al, 2001) – especially when work was included in the mix. Greenwood (2002: 127) confirms that action researchers delve into life 'messes': complex, dynamic and difficult problems, such as those presented here (Vickers, 2005e).

An insider-outsider perspective

A critical feature of action research is the involvement and input of the researcher in the process. The researcher feeds back the findings to participants along the way so that they have input on what happens next (Page and Meyer, 2000: 20). Action researchers are required to be both inside and outside the research and social change process; to be engaged in it, and to reflect on the process, before, during and after action (Fricke, 2004). Action research is insider-outsider and multiparty work (Greenwood, 2002: 127).

I was both inside and outside the phenomenon under review (Vickers, 2005e), in several material ways. First, I was inside the phenomenon because I worked full-time. I was also a *woman* working full-time, with all the careerist and gender issues that this implied. Secondly, I had been the carer of a person (my partner) with a significant chronic illness. His condition had prompted his disability-related retirement from a banking career at the age of 43. I saw his illness rampage through our lives and witnessed, not just his physical and emotional loss and suffering, but mine. I understood the grief and loss associated with serious illness. I had also lived the uncertainty, change, inconvenience, and fear associated with caring for another, as well as the absence of understanding, consideration and support from others. I had learned that illness and disability could undermine relationships, shift interpersonal dynamics, induce financial hardship, and initiate unanticipated struggle, ambivalence and turmoil (Vickers, 2005e).

Finally, I was also a person with a significant chronic illness myself: I have multiple sclerosis. I understood the vagaries and uncertainties of chronic illness first-hand. I understood the discrimination, stigma, alienation, fear, loss and grief that chronic illness could bring, and I was very familiar with the unpredictable mural a life with chronic illness portrays, especially as it reaches into the future (Vickers, 2005e). I had coped with varying levels of disability – visible and invisible – over many years, and in concert with working and living. However, concurrently, I had learned the growth possible from surviving, and the strength and fearlessness that accompanies successful encounters with adversity. I appreciated the joy and richness life can bring, even when trouble strikes. For this study, it was imperative, then, that these 'inside' perspectives be enabled and acknowledged. I was, in so many ways, researching from the inside (Vickers, 2002a).

However, in other important ways, I was on the outside, looking in. I had no children, so had little understanding of parenting, especially the mother-child bond, the selfless caring that accompanies parenthood, or the need to juggle work and home with children thrown into the time-hungry mix. I also professed no knowledge of the special grief and loss engendered by having a child with chronic illness, nor the fears for the future felt for a child more vulnerable than most. My concurrent proximity and distance to this research was undeniable (Vickers, 2005e). According to Heidegger, the researcher's influence cannot be underestimated and will determine what phenomena, facts and relations enter their consciousness (Moss and Keen, 1981: 108). The researcher's orientation, sensitivity and perceptiveness shape the interpretations (Osborne, 1990: 85; Vickers, 2001a).

I was also both inside and outside the process of *doing* the research (Vickers, 2005e). I was inside the research as a researcher sharing a journey with my respondents, unclear what was around the next corner, but anxious to know. However, I was also outside the process. I was not a participant in this study. In response to this ambiguous place, you will find my researcher reflections peppered throughout this volume. I was acutely aware that I did not wish to place my insights, fears and highlights outside the reported outcomes. My confessionals of this methodological adventure – not always comfortable – have not been relegated to appendices, footnotes and introductory comments because I did not want them to merely supplement the 'real story' (Kleinman and Copp, 1993: 17). While my initial leaning was to place them as footnotes along the way – to be witnessed *alongside* the other accounts, while not distracting from them – I have, instead, placed them throughout the chapters, among respondent stories, as an adjunct to other interpretive, descriptive and explanatory text. I have termed them Researcher Notes. You will see that, sometimes, I was comfortable with what I was doing and what these women were telling me; at other times I was not. Sometimes I felt very unsure; at other times, I understood *exactly* what was said.

A unique research design

The important connection between theory and action – social praxis – is demonstrated through the dialogues between researchers and subjects (Fricke, 2004). Certainly, the respondents in this project were subjects (rather than objects) and it is hoped that, in the pages that follow, evidence of the 'field talking back' will become clear (Fricke, 2004). At all stages of the project, respondents were encouraged to participate (although, because of their particular circumstances, not all were able to, all the time). Certainly, I viewed participants as equal, bowing to their vastly greater knowledge of their experiences on one hand, and choosing to retain my researcher-imbued authority over data selection, presentation and choices on the other.

Action research projects attempt to make change, and to gather and analyse data concurrently (Punch, 1998). The focus is on the applied nature of the social research and upon taking action as a result of the findings; to effect ongoing change (Page and Meyer, 2000: 20). Action research requires the mobilisation of expertise from any and all academic and research locations that are relevant, and any research methods can be relevant insofar as they have something specific to contribute (Greenwood, 2002: 127). The creation of fruitful and mutually beneficial interaction between actionable knowledge and textual knowledge is no small task (Palshaugen, 2004a: 113). This project embraced, with care, several philosophical and methodological choices, and the research design consisted of several distinct stages:

Stage 1: **In-depth Interviews:** *Retrospective* Perspective; Heideggerian Phenomenology.

Stage 2: **In-depth Interviews:** *Prospective* Perspective; Clarification of Data; Responses to Vignettes; Heideggerian Phenomenology and Naturalistic Inquiry; Actionable Knowledge and Change.

Stage 3: **Culminating Group Experience (CGE):** Naturalistic Inquiry; Member Checking; Actionable Knowledge and Change. (Vickers, 2005c: 206; 2005e: 197)

For this exploratory, qualitative study, only a small number of participants were interviewed. Nine women[2] who had lived (or were living) the phenomenon under investigation participated with final numbers remaining small because: (1) the study was exploratory; (2) smaller numbers of participants allowed for more penetrating insights where the quantity of data collected can become overwhelming; and, (3) the study was designed to test the research design methodologically and substantively. I had not previously used naturalistic inquiry, nor had I found another who had used it in combination with Heideggerian phenomenology, or action research, nor employing the specific methods undertaken here.

Methodologically, I wanted to learn: (1) how well the use of retrospective and prospective interviewing worked; (2) how useful the fictional vignettes were; and, (3) whether the CGE achieved its aims. Substantively, I was concerned with: (1) how well the methods utilised provided the data sought; and, (2) whether the data gathered answered the research question. I will return to these concerns in Chapter 8.

Purposive sampling was used to recruit participants (see Vickers, 2001a; Baird, 2003):

1. Respondents could be male or female;
2. Respondents must be in full-time employment (or equivalent), or have been in full-time employment during the last 12 months;
3. Respondents must have (or have had) primary caring or parental responsibility (which may be shared with a live-in partner) for a child with chronic illness (as defined in Chapter 1).

The interpretivist paradigm was chosen for this research project. Interpretivist researchers work from the standpoint that people experience physical and social reality in different ways. These meaning systems, or patterns of conventions, are created out of social interactions. Reality is considered to be socially constructed (Berger and Luckmann, 1966; Gergen and Gergen, 1984; Shotter, 1989; Harris, Trezise and Winser, 2002). Interpretive research takes everyday experience and ordinary life as its subject matter and asks how meaning is constructed and social interaction negotiated in social practices (Scott and Usher, 1999: 25; Green, 2002: 6). I was interested in understanding the lived experience of these people and remained concerned about reporting their experiences, through their eyes, and understanding the meaning it held for them (Vickers, 2005e).

Respondents were recruited via a word-of-mouth, modified chain referral technique. Success has been experienced elsewhere with this recruitment technique, especially given the small sample size and the sensitive nature of what was being investigated. This approach was successfully adopted by Watters and Biernacki (1989) and, later, myself

(Vickers, 1997a; 2001a). 'Intermediaries' were asked to contact potentially eligible participants: colleagues, friends, and family were approached to ask if they knew anyone who might be a likely candidate for participation. In this way, the intermediary (rather than the researcher) could make the first contact with the potential respondent. Information sheets and consent forms were also made available to respondents. Once interviews commenced, respondents were also asked for possible further referrals for others who may have been available to participate in this study.

Researcher Note: *Actually, in several instances, I didn't even have to ask. Respondents routinely volunteered to contact people on my behalf to be included in the study. Indeed, I found that whenever I spoke with anyone about my study, they told me that they knew someone who could potentially participate. Referrals were not hard to find. As the first round of interviews drew to a close, I had to actually ask one person not to contact their friend, as I had enough data to proceed to Stage Two* (Vickers, Researcher Reflections, Friday, 5 December 2003).

Data from all three stages of the project were utilised to share these women's experiences and is depicted variously via extracted narratives from respondents, researcher notes and reflections, and data poems created by the researcher using the words of respondents (Moisiewicz, 2005). Fictional diary entries were also composed – drawing on the various experiences shared by respondents (Vallant, 2005) – to represent a typical 'day in the life' of a fictional mother of a child with a chronic illness. The first of these is found in the Introduction to this volume; the second – intended as a rebuttal to the first – is reported in the Epilogue. Finally, fictional vignettes were developed, also from data gathered, to elicit further responses to likely scenarios.

The purpose of all these varied narrative inclusions was that it allowed me to better 'show, not tell' what life was like for these women. Certainly, my interpretations were included, but I wanted readers to grasp these women's reality: to feel it; to see it in their mind's eye; to live it. I wanted readers to also have their eyes shine with tears; to feel provoked, angry, frustrated, and shocked. I wanted readers to know these women's lives. Like Sandelowski (1994: 46), I was trying to convey the ideas, with artfulness not being considered a fault. Sandelowski refutes the idea that being artful is somehow not being faithful to your data: 'art and science are not necessarily two

distinct things' (Sandelowski, 1994: 46). She likens the process to one
of working clay on a potter's wheel. I loved the analogy:

> The pot carries its maker's thoughts, feelings, and spirit. To overlook
> this fact is to miss a crucial truth, whether in clay, story, or science
> (Krieger, 1991: 89; cited in Sandelowski, 1994: 47).

So, like Sandelowski, I refused to 'refuse the art', while doing my best
to practice intellectual craftsmanship (Mills, 1959: 195) when writing
and presenting the data. Celebrating, rather than refusing, the art per-
mitted me to present these women's lives in a manner that would get
attention; that would get them a hearing so that something might be
done. According to Cross (1990: 193), without this, I would have just
remained a 'fact grubber' and a 'rule follower'. Not for me, and not for
these women.

The basis of this project was the experiences of respondents (Fricke,
2004), my desire to share those experiences with others (Vickers,
2001a), and the fact that, from the outset, the project was driven by a
problem about which not enough was known. The data shared in this
chapter is used to portray how data from each stage was used as the
project evolved, to demonstrate the knowledge gained along the way,
and the actionable knowledge outcomes that resulted. The 'theory'
that emerged (and reported in subsequent chapters) was developed in
conjunction with participants, within their social context, and as a
result of joint learning by both researcher and participants (Fricke,
2004).

Doing the research: how it worked

In this section, I will discuss each of the three stages of the project,
including how the philosophical and methodological choices made
influenced the data gathering and data gathered. Fricke (2004) reminds
us that action researchers must be able to use a toolkit of different
methods, and be especially competent in the areas of value orientation,
empathy, and responsibility for the consequences of their research. I
approached the field with a desire to learn, to view experiences
through the eyes of my respondents, to enter into a dialogue with
them, and to develop useful knowledge of the situation and contextual
theory as part of a process of action and reflection (Fricke, 2004). I
shared Dick's view that action research should be carefully considered,
rigorous and high quality, while also agreeing that each single case can

have a useful contribution to make (Dick, 2003: 256). This study involved nine respondents in Stage 1; six in Stage 2; and two in Stage 3 (Vickers, 2005e). The exploratory nature of the study encouraged and enabled learning from both experience and theory (that is, understanding from past practice) (Dick, 2003: 256).

Stage 1: In-depth interviews

Purpose: Retrospective perspective;
Philosophy: Heideggerian phenomenology.

I sought to retain the fundamental essence of the phenomenological purpose in this first stage. I had worked extensively with Heideggerian phenomenology in the past (see Vickers, 2001a), so I understood that Heideggerian phenomenology did not require me to 'bracket' my knowledge or experience, as would be required for either Husserlian phenomenology or, other more positivistic approaches. This orientation also centred around the need to capture the subjectively experienced life of the informants as interpreted by them (Taylor, 1993: 174), describing the respondents' lived experience (Oiler, 1982: 178) and the meaning it held for them (Drew, 1989: 431; Vickers, 2001a: 33) – capturing the richness of individual experience (Baker, Wuest and Stern, 1992: 1358; Vickers, 2001a: 33). I also knew that Heideggerian phenomenology valued an acceptance of multiplicity in people's lives and experiences (Taylor, 1993: 174; Vickers, 2001a; 2005e). In this study, the women demonstrated multiple, overlapping and conflicting lives, roles and identities. Heideggerian phenomenology allowed for a composite of realities (Oiler, 1982: 179; Gergen and Gergen, 1984: 182; Bateson, 1989: 162; Gergen, 1991: 83; Davis, 1994: 353; Vickers, 2005e).

Heideggerian phenomenology also allowed me to value my proximity to the study at hand. Interviews encouraging discussion, sharing of experiences, and *retrospective* reflections were conducted. Respondents were asked: What happened? How did you feel? What did you do? Why did you take that action? Of primary concern was learning their concerns and the meaning it held for them, as they reflected on what had gone before (Vickers, 2005e). Respondents were asked a series of open-ended questions that were intended specifically to explore complex, often very personal matters (Alvesson, 2003: 19). The focus areas for interviews shifted as the interviews and project progressed. Intensive interpretation was required, before, during and after the interview, to form some assumptions about these women's lives, although it was recognised that these assumptions would rarely be explicit. These interpretive processes were really what the entire exercise was about (Alvesson, 2003: 19).

What follows is an example of data drawn from Stage 1. Readers will recall having been introduced to Dolly, who lived with her intellectually disabled daughter who also suffered from severe epilepsy. Dolly had recently separated from her husband. Dolly's mother, who had previously been living with Dolly and her husband and providing after-school care for Maggie, had just moved out after an argument with Dolly. At the time of our first meeting, Dolly was on her own, caring for her disabled child and working full-time. She described her multiple and conflicting roles, multiple identities and her experience of 'doing it all' (explored further in Chapter 3) (Vickers, Parris and Bailey, 2004; Vickers and Parris, 2005):

> **Dolly:** What [Steven] doesn't understand is, yes, he takes Margaret three weekends out of four. But who organises all Maggie's medication, organises all her doctor's appointments? Who takes her to all her blood tests? Who irons all her clothes? Who washes all her clothes? Who changes all her bed? Who organises all the nappies? This all just happens. Who buys all her clothes? Who finds time to go and buy her clothes and get her shoes fitted? And this all happens around Steven, and he doesn't *get it*. Who does all the grocery shopping? You know, the food is just there; the clothes are there. She goes with a perfect little bag, like an overnight bag, with all the medication, all the stuff. And I'm really filthy with him, because it all comes back dirty. And I said to him, you know, 'You can *wash*. You know, it would be really good, you've got her from Friday night to Sunday night, you can wash … I don't expect two or three sets of pyjamas to come back filthy'. You know, because Maggie's a bit of a grub. 'You know, it wouldn't hurt you to do a wash and all that sort of thing'. So, hopefully he will do that. (Dolly, Interview 1: 36; Vickers, Parris and Bailey, 2004: 41; Vickers and Parris, 2005: 100)

Dolly was sharing her personal experience of having to 'do it all', reflecting on her past experiences from a retrospective perspective, telling me what *had happened*, how she *had felt* and *what her response had been* to those circumstances. I was able to see, through her eyes, what this experience was for her. I learned about Dolly's multiple roles, the time she needed, and how angry and frustrated she was when her husband didn't wash the dirty linen.

Researcher Note: *As a career woman with little time to spare myself, I could readily understand her anger. As a chronically ill person and carer of a loved one, the obvious lack of support she experienced also resonated with me – hence the likely reason for my choice of this passage for inclusion, rather than another, to make this point. I also empathised with her efforts to manage her multiple, and often conflicting roles and identities: She was a mother, HR professional, ex-wife, carer, negotiator, and daughter; I was an academic, person with multiple sclerosis, researcher, author, wife, carer, and daughter. I wondered how she coped with her overlapping realities and conflicting responsibilities. I knew it had been hard for me. At times, when my partner was very sick, I remembered feeling completely overwhelmed, wondering how I would keep going. I heard this from Dolly. As I reflected on all this, I was reminded of my responsibility to share Dolly's story (and those of the other women interviewed), to understand it as best I could, and to do something to help them and those similarly placed, if I could.* (Vickers, Researcher Reflections, Wednesday, 14 May 2003; Vickers, 2005e: 200)

Prior to moving to Stage 2 where I reinterviewed respondents, I reviewed the transcripts of interviews from Stage 1 for the specific purpose of developing questions from a *prospective* perspective and to clarify any possible misunderstanding that I might have formed. Aside from further exploring and developing certain themes, I wanted to ask: If you had your time over, what would change? What will you do differently in the future? I also developed a number of fictional vignettes for presentation to respondents during that second interview. These fictional vignettes were mostly based on data gathered from Stage 1 (see Appendix).

Stage 2: In-depth interviews

Purpose: Prospective perspective; clarification of data; responses to fictional vignettes;
Philosophy: Heideggerian phenomenology and naturalistic inquiry;[3] actionable knowledge and change.

One of the tenets of naturalistic inquiry is to gather data from multiple sources for triangulation (Lincoln and Guba, 1985; Erlandson et al, 1993: 31; Harris, Trezise and Winser, 2002: 11). However, naturalistic inquiry similarly recognises the need for a window of meaning on lives where multiple realities can be revealed through thick description (Green, 2002: 14). Indeed, the post-positivist paradigm proposes a reality where all aspects of reality are interrelated. The assumption is that to isolate one aspect from its context destroys much of its meaning (Vickers, 2005e). Naturalistic inquiry assumes no single objective reality, but multiple realities that individual perspectives give rise to (Harris, Trezise and Winser, 2002; Erlandson et al, 1993: 14).

Many of the tenets of Heideggerian phenomenology and naturalistic inquiry also overlapped. For example, the key elements of naturalistic inquiry included many elements also used in Heideggerian phenomenology: the use of the human being as an instrument; tacit knowledge; qualitative methods; purposive sampling; inductive data analysis; the case report; thick description; idiographic interpretation; and trustworthiness (Lincoln and Guba, 1985; Green, 2002: 8; Vickers, 2005e).[4]

The focus on context is also viewed as holding the key to all meaning (Lincoln and Guba, 1985; Erlandson et al, 1993: 16; Green, 2002: 5). The context of this study was not a physical or social one.[5] Here, instead, two concurrent contextual dynamics were involved: first, the need to manage substantial caring responsibilities with the continual demands of full-time work; secondly, to manage full-time work with the continuing backdrop of parental caring responsibilities. It was the continual entanglement of full-time work with caring responsibilities that presented the dilemmas and experiences that seeped into all areas of their lives: their financial standing, careers, self, and relationships with family, friends, children and partners (Vickers, 2005e). Complex and interwoven concepts necessitated a holistic approach to inquiry (Glesne and Peshkin, 1992; Harris, Trezise and Winser, 2002). The best way to elicit the various and divergent constructions of reality that exist within the context of a study is to collect information about different events and relationships from different points of view (Erlandson et al, 1993: 31). For example, Mason (2001) included two rounds of interviews, group discussions and individually written outcomes (Mason, 2001: 311–312). I followed Mason's example, believing that the model of several stages and different modes of data gathering would contribute to a richer understanding.

Using naturalistic inquiry also enabled me to consider my 'insider-outsider' status. Henderson et al's (2002) naturalistic inquiry of young children's literacy also utilised the insider-researcher and outsider-researcher perspectives to great effect (Henderson et al, 2002: 309). Finally, naturalistic inquiry, like Heideggerian phenomenology, brought recognition of the need for a window of meaning on lives where multiple realities could be revealed through thick description (Green, 2002: 14).

Prospective perspective; clarification and data: Stage 2 interviews were designed to clarify or further explore issues raised in the Stage 1 interviews. Transcription and early analysis was undertaken between interviews, and emergent themes further explored and uncertainties remedied. For example, when I returned to the second interview with Dolly, I asked her more about her situation of 'doing it all'. Dolly had told me in the first interview that she rarely had an unbroken night's sleep because her daughter still had regular night seizures, or was wakeful and restless. Dolly reported having to get up at night to attend to her child (as there was no-one else) and still going to work the next day.

Researcher Note: *The problem of Dolly not being able to get regular sleep resonated with me enormously. As one with a chronic condition myself, managing a full-time job alongside my own chronic illness is a constant challenge. Energy, for me, is a most precious commodity. As I listened to Dolly, I was trying to imagine how on earth I would be able function if, every night, I was unable to get sufficient sleep. I could not see how I could do it. I just could not imagine how one could function, especially in the senior role that Dolly had, in any way that was not simply a constant, miserable struggle. I wanted to hear more about this.*
(Vickers, Researcher Reflections, Wednesday, 16 April 2003)

I explored Dolly's sense of feeling overwhelmed and having to 'do it all' by asking her what she might do in the future:

Researcher: You also spoke last time about your concerns about feeling overwhelmed, that it's 'all you' in terms of coping with Margaret. You expressed concerns about not being able to continue doing it all in the future. What sort of things might help with this situation, for you?
Dolly: Well, probably at the time, I don't know that I had the other carers in place. So I think having a bigger network, for me, is impor-tant ... I feel that it's a bit bigger now, and it probably wouldn't hurt to actually try to increase that again somehow, I don't know. I think that's an opportunity thing. I've got to go to mothers' groups or school groups or something like that – which I haven't actually got time to do – to sort of create those opportunities. My problem with some of those groups is that they usually work on a pay-back system – 'I'll look after yours and you look after mine'. I can't promise to look after someone. So it's going to be more that I can just add more

people to my minding pile, if I need to. (Dolly, Interview 2: 15–16; Vickers, 2005e: 203)

In this extract, we see the shift to the *prospective* perspective. While learning more about Dolly's experience of 'doing it all', I could see further evidence of her multiple lives, multiple roles and multiple identities. However, also presented was evidence of changes in her behaviour and thinking as a result of the research process. She spoke of needing to get further child minding assistance. She also, poignantly, highlighted her disconnectedness (explored further in Chapter 3) with the other mothers of children with chronic illness. As Dolly explained, she just could not work with them on the 'pay-back' system because she had to work. In Dolly's account of 'doing it all', learning was taking place and changes to her behaviour and thinking were evident. Dolly confirmed her actionable knowledge as she spoke of putting herself 'back on the list':

> **Researcher:** If you had your time over, would you do anything differently?
> **Dolly:** Absolutely. I'd put myself back on the list. Because I think, by not looking after myself, physically, emotionally, spiritually, I think that's brought a whole lot of the other things undone in my life. I think it's been a contributing factor to a whole bunch of stuff that I could have managed better; I could have managed my mother better, I could have managed my husband better. I would have felt a lot better. I wouldn't have put on five or six stone. I would have felt a lot more positive about who I was, and a bit more in control. So, yes, if I knew what I know now, I would definitely have done things differently. (Dolly, Interview 2: 8; Vickers, 2005e: 205)

Action researchers confirm that the only meaningful way to theorise is through successive cycles of combined reflection and action, the action feeding back to revise the reflection in ongoing cycles (Greenwood, 2002: 125). Dolly had reflected on her experiences and learned to do things differently in the future.

Responses to Vignettes: Participants in Stage 2 were also presented with case study vignettes that had been developed as a result of the data gathered from Stage 1. Vignettes focused on difficulties, reported or anticipated, such as: not being able to apply for a particular job; ongoing loss and grief; anxiety surrounding the development of new (partner) relationships; support received or not received; childcare concerns; 'family-friendly' policies in workplaces; responses to emergencies, especially while at work; disguising child-related concerns in the work context; insufficient knowledge of support services and financial assistance; and questions of disclosure related to their child, especially at work.

Researcher Note: *The respondents' experiences from Stage 1 are providing brilliant and direct input into the development of the fictional vignettes. I will also be using my hunches, ideas gathered from the literature, but the 'real feel' that I can offer respondents by using these vignettes based on reality seems very powerful. Stories like Cate's leap to the foreground. I am wondering just what their response will be.* (Vickers, Researcher Reflections, Monday, 9 June 2003)

I found it very useful to tell respondents, during the Stage 2 interviews, that the fictional vignettes offered to them were based on real life examples. This added a degree of 'authenticity' that I believed influenced the responses. In total, 14 vignettes were developed (see Appendix). Several of these were presented to participants during Stage 2. Vignettes based on a respondent's own experiences were not given to them for comment, although I did direct certain vignettes to people I thought might relate to a particular scenario.

Vignettes ranged from a short paragraph, to scenarios involving several separate, short sections, with questions being asked at specific cues along the way. I share here an example of data from Stage 1 which provided input into one of the vignettes. Readers are reminded that Cate worked full-time, had a four-year-old son with autism, a disabled adult brother living with her, a husband who didn't appear to work or assist with home duties in any meaningful way, and another two-year-old dependent child to care for. She shared this compelling anecdote, which was preceded by her poignant comments that she didn't trust her husband alone with her autistic son for any length of time:

Cate: It was a day when the kids were home because it was Christmas Eve. The kids were home, no daycare. I had to work but I was going to come home early. I said, 'I'm coming home early. You've got to watch the kids, but don't worry because I'll be home early'. And so I went home, and it was about two in the afternoon, and his car was not there. And I went inside and guess who's there? The two kids – alone ... And I was, 'What is going on?' They were just sitting in the living room, but you can't leave a two-year-old

and a four-year-old home alone ... and then about 40 minutes later
he shows up – with alcohol. You know, he's got alcohol. He was
already alcoholed up. He was already shit-faced [drunk]. (Cate,
Interview 1: 21–22; Vickers, Parris and Bailey, 2004: 41–42; Vickers,
2005e: 207)

Thus, Vignette 10 was inspired by Cate's experience (and also
Dolly's):

Vignette 10: Childcare concerns

You have had considerable difficulty finding someone to look
after your child during school holidays, and to be there after
school when your child arrives home, around 3 pm. However,
you find this person in the local paper. They have references and
appear knowledgeable (well, a bit) about your child's illness.
They are confident with the child, and tell you they have
worked as a nurse's aid at a hospital some years ago.

On this particular day, you arrive home from work early. You
have just got a promotion and decided to give yourself a reward
by taking the rest of the afternoon off. You arrive home and find
your child sitting in front of the television in a dirty nappy. This
is not just any dirty nappy. It should have been changed many
hours ago.

Where is your carer? Nowhere to be seen. You notice – for the
first time since she started work – a dirty ashtray, full of cigarette butts. You recall asking her if she smoked when you
interviewed her for the job, because you didn't want cigarette
smoke around your child. She had said no.

About 20 minutes later, the carer arrives home, sees you
and is very apologetic. She tells you that she just *had* to get
some cigarettes down at the local shop and was only a few
moments.

It is Friday, and next week is school holidays. What do you
do? How do you feel? What are you most concerned about –
now and in the future? (Vignette 10, Appendix; Vickers, 2005e:
207–208)

Evalyn was asked to respond to this vignette. Unlike Cate, Evalyn
had reported a supportive partner relationship. However, Evalyn had
also expressed her concerns in finding suitable carers for her child. Her
response was this:

Evalyn: Oh, this is a difficult one. I wouldn't be happy... I would not be happy.

Researcher: Which particular issues would make you unhappy?

Evalyn: The most serious issue is leaving my child alone. I can't really have a carer that smokes around my child, and I'm not really excited about it; I don't like it ... But I'd rather have a caring carer than a nonsmoking, noncaring carer. Smoking really wouldn't, I don't like it but it's not something that I would sort of see as a big determinant in whether someone is a good carer or not. But a dirty nappy – okay. That's not my situation and obviously is a sign of neglect. But the *really serious* neglect was the fact that she left my child *alone* for *who knows how long!* And that's serious. That's not good enough. I could not, in good conscience, allow that carer to look after my child – absolutely not! That's just not acceptable, leaving my child alone. If it was leaving my child alone and going to bring the clothes in, okay, I could understand that, because it's just going out to get the clothes in. But leaving my child alone to go and buy cigarettes – which is, I don't know how far away – that's *appalling* [incredulous]. Okay, it's extremely disruptive because next week it's school holidays, but I'm going to have to let this carer go. I'd feel absolutely appalled. Just devastated that I, I'd be really upset about this thing. I'd ring the referees and tell them off. Concerned about now? Of course, I'd be very concerned about the future because it's not easy finding carers who are supposed to be experienced, but I'd just have to get around it and ring my mum up [laughter]. (Evalyn, Interview 2: 16–17; Vickers, 2005e: 209)

Researcher Note: *I have a comment to make regarding my 'insider-outsider' status. As I review what Evalyn says about this situation, I really feel lacking. I have no idea about caring for a child, let alone finding carers for them, especially one with special needs. I was quite concerned, when I developed this vignette, that I had the details (especially surrounding nappy changing, etc) reasonably plausible. I was very relieved that Evalyn's response indicated that my vignette captured the situation as I had intended. Then I thought about it: who could I have called on if placed in a similar situation? I have never called a babysitter in my life. Do I have close friends I could rely on for this? Would my mother (who is now well into her seventies) be prepared to do this? Would my sister? I had to reluctantly consider the possibility that I would, like Cate (whose experience the vignette was based on) really have little support also if I was thrust into this kind of situation. Certainly, if I had children, I would* *know other people, possibly have other friends that I might have been able to call on. But this was a discomforting acknowledgement, all the same. Had I ever babysat my own sister's children? No. My brother's? No. I had looked after a couple of close girlfriends' children (with no chronic illness or special needs) for a couple of very short periods, but had found the experience nothing short of terrifying – such a responsibility! Yes, my definite lack of knowledge and experience in this area left me feeling very uncertain. That said, it also got me thinking about these women's lives in a way that I never had before.* (Vickers, Researcher Reflections, Thursday, 16 October 2003)

Evalyn shared her feelings of grave concern – even fear – that a carer might leave her disabled son alone for any period of time. This was certainly an issue that required more research. Evalyn also highlighted the difficulty that many of the mothers noted in being able to get quality carers for their child, especially at short notice. Finally, I noted that it was Evalyn, not her partner, who would have been organising the new carer.

Researcher Note: *I am certain that Cate probably shared all of these concerns too. But I also knew that, for her, this wasn't just any carer who had been irresponsible – it was her husband. And I also knew that Cate's mother (as you will see in Chapter 5) was also not available for backup, or emergency situations as Evalyn's was. Cate's lack of support is becoming more and more pronounced in my mind.* (Vickers, Researcher Reflections, Friday, 6 May, 2005)

Stage 3: Culminating group experience (CGE)

Purpose: Member checking;
Philosophy: Naturalistic inquiry; member checking; actionable knowledge and change.

The CGE was not run as a traditional focus group. Instead, the trustworthiness of the findings was being checked, as was further evidence of learning or behaviour change as a result of the research process, specifically at the local level. The session was also taped and transcribed, offering further data (Vickers, 2005e). Many studies using naturalistic inquiry gather data from multiple sources for triangulation (Lincoln and Guba, 1985; Erlandson et al, 1993: 31; Harris, Trezise and Winser, 2002: 11). The aim was to collect information about different events and relationships from different points of view (Erlandson et al,

1993: 31). A period of two months was deliberately interspersed after the conclusion of Stage 2 giving me time to consider early themes and issues of concern to present to respondents. The schedule was this:

4.15–4.30 pm	*Welcome and drinks*
4.30–5.30 pm	*Presentation of Preliminary Findings and Proposed Future Research*
5.30–6.00 pm	*Group Discussion: Research Process Review*
6.00–6.30 pm	*Group Discussion and Network Opportunity: Where to Now?*
6.30 pm	*Close*

I discussed and presented my provisional and emerging findings, and some of the responses to the fictional vignettes. I hoped to: (1) generate discussion; (2) learn of the accuracy or otherwise of my interpretations; (3) learn about the respondents' experience of participating in the research; and, (4) provide opportunities for respondents to network with one another. While their participation was still anonymous (participants were allocated and referred to by number that evening), they could choose to disclose their names and details to anyone else, as they wished. Finishing the project with this group experience also allowed a sense of closure. Readers may be concerned that there was a substantial drop off in numbers as the project proceeded. Stage 1 included nine respondents; Stage 2 included six[6] respondents. Stage 3 included just two respondents.[7] However, Stage 3 did achieve its set objectives, and provided material evidence of actionable knowledge outcomes.

Research Note: *During the presentation, I became very aware of the response of the two women who were participating. They were listening very carefully. There were no questions, at all, during my presentation. At one point, I could see one respondent working hard to hold back her tears; sadness was in the room. I was able to see this clearly from where I stood talking to them. I was also nervous. I had never before during a project 'fed back' my interpretations to respondents for comment. What if I was wrong? What if I had completely misunderstood, or missed something very important to them altogether? It was an uncomfortable forum for me – but one that I wouldn't have missed for the world. The feedback was not only encouraging and invigorating, but left me feeling good about what I had been doing. I felt that they were telling me that they were being 'heard' for the first time; that someone out there cared about their lives* *and their lot. I was relieved and delighted. They also reported a positive experience from participating in the research; I hadn't anticipated that. Finally, they gave me feedback on my interpretations that helped me further develop my thoughts about what was emerging, confirming some areas, and highlighting the strength of others that were less obvious to me.* (Vickers, Researcher Reflections, Monday, 24 November 2003)

Learning from respondents was evident via their comments about their participation in the project, their responses to the data presented, and subsequent discussion. Wendy shared her reflections on the theme of 'doing it all', drawing another issue of concern to the fore – the lack of knowledge that other people have of these women's plight:

> **Wendy:** I've just been thinking, one of the things that struck me is it's like housework. It's invisible. And the theme of invisibility. And then, just then, if you go: women's housework, women's mothering and caring, and *then* the carer of the disabled or ill, it's the triple-load; it's not the double workload, it's the triple-load. You have the triple bottom line in business; you have the triple bottom load. It's not a double whammy; it's an extra one. (Wendy, CGE: 3; Vickers, 2005e: 210)

> **Researcher Note:** *Wendy's comment sums it all up for me. This was originally the whole reason for doing this project: to draw attention to a problem that was currently neglected. Wendy bringing this out, so pointedly, in this final session and after hearing my exploratory themes, reminded me of those original concerns that had prompted the study in the first place. I was relieved to be on the right track.* (Vickers, Researcher Reflections, Friday, 6 May 2005)

I also saw Wendy's learning from the research process. She specifically pointed out that she had begun to act upon her own needs since participating in the project. She shared how she had been able to 'hand over' a small part of the responsibilities relating to her child's care to her daughter's father. This, she explained, involved recognition by him of the mental and physical activities involved:

> **Wendy:** We have to do a monthly trip down to Sydney to pick up medication. And I've now got to the point of having been able to train my kid's father to go and do that. And he's moved from going and collecting it when we ring up and check it is in the pharmacy

and all of that. He's now moved to: 'What are you going to do when you're away and you need the second one? You'd better ring the doctor and get a double dose'. And I'm handing it back. It's like: 'Talk to your dad and make sure that he has enough scripts'. So I'm managing it more and more remotely, so that now not only does he pay the monthly prescription cost, but he also goes and picks it up, anticipates it. He throws his little 'wobblies' when it's not there, and rings me up in meetings and tells me, 'What am I going to do about it?' And I just say, 'Sorry, I'm in a meeting. Bye, bye!' [Laughter] You know, it's that invisible 'packing the bag' [referring to Dolly's earlier comments from Stage 1] and all of that.

Researcher: But you've had to manage it back to your partner too; it hasn't just happened. You've had to figure out, 'How am I going to do this?' And you've got your daughter to do this.

Wendy: That's right. And that's only a tiny little bit.

Researcher: *I know.* That's just one little bit.

Wendy: That's once monthly, that's four hours a month. That's half a day a month, but that's quite considerable for me. (Wendy, CGE: 15; Vickers, 2005e: 211)

Part II
Acknowledging the Anguish

3
Disconnected and Doing it All

It's All Me

Wondering whether I'm going to cope
I don't know
A child with a disability –
I want to have a life.

Hard to connect
She's in her own little world.
Cuddles and kisses and chasings –
Only so much I can do.

Would she be better off with him?
Is he better equipped?
He's with a partner.
It *is* hard looking after a child like that.

My ability to sustain –
Am I actually built that way?
It's all me now. It's all me.
Am I really up for it?

(Dolly, Interview 1: 28–29)

The data poem created from Dolly's words captures the uncertainty
and feelings of being overwhelmed that these women often spoke of,
especially as they juggled their many roles and responsibilities. This
chapter depicts respondents having to do it all. In Chapter 1, we
learned that women continue to do a great deal of work – often much
more than men – that is diffused between their job, household, and
childcare responsibilities. Depending on the specific nature of their

paid and unpaid work responsibilities, we know that women's work-loads can contribute to mental and physical health problems, marital stress, career interruptions or reduced work hours, and lower job status (Gjerdingen et al, 2000: 15). Women are, generally, struggling with multiple roles – that overlap and conflict – that predispose them to high levels of role strain and occupational stress (see Chapter 1).

For women who also care for a child with a chronic condition, the burden is worse; the pressure harder to bear; the roles more complex. The result? Women feeling disconnected, overwhelmed, and alone – women 'doing it all'. I explore here two key themes that emerged from these women's stories and reflections:

- Feeling disconnected; and,
- Doing it all.

Feeling disconnected

The women in this study all reported their tremendous struggle balancing work and home life, especially with the enormous physical and emotional burdens placed upon them as a result of their caring responsibilities (Vickers and Bailey, 2003; Vickers, Bailey and Parris, 2003; Vickers, Parris and Bailey, 2004). All reported, in one way or another, feeling different, disconnected or apart from those they worked with and related to; that others did not really understand their lives.

Part of this sense of 'otherness' was feeling alone. Fromm (1942/1960: 23; Vickers, 2001a: 101) spoke of the likelihood of 'growing aloneness' increasing in an individualist culture – which is where these women were situated. As Fromm (1942/1960: 23) reminds us: 'when one has become an individual, one stands alone and faces the world in all its perilous and overpowering consequences'. For these women, standing alone was reflected in their obvious need for, and others' inadequate response to, support, both formal and informal. Many authors have highlighted the need to tailor specific support programs to the expressed needs of family carers, with a view to improving the quality of life of those individuals (Chambers, Ryan and Connor, 2001: 100). Indeed, social support is a resource that we know can influence the extent to which stressful situations, such as those associated with major caring responsibilities, influence psychological well-being (Chambers, Ryan and Connor, 2001: 100). We also know that family caregivers provide a vital and increasing service to society, and yet little help is offered to support them as they struggle to fulfil their roles (McGrath, 2001: 199). Sadly, studies have shown that carers often have little emotional support, and report feeling abandoned; that there is no-one 'out there' to help or that understands them. Loneliness and isolation are key concerns (Chambers, Ryan and Connor, 2001: 101) as is the ability to lead a normal life (Knafl and Deatrick, 2002).

The enormity of these women's challenge and their sense of being overwhelmed at every turn underlined much of their daily life. Jack's (1991) work is based on the belief that the behaviours of women are affected by social learning. Women learn not to express what they need and feel openly and directly (DeMarco, Lynch and Board, 2002: 90). There were many parallels reported here, such as the problematic role of gender norms (Jack, 1991: 14), a loss of voice, especially in partner relationships (Jack, 1991: 30), and the perceived need to silence the self. However, also reported were distinctions from Jack's (1991) theory, that draw attention to current gender debates about the work-home conflict, and the stresses attaching to informal care provision; both issues that require further attention, debate and action (Vickers and Parris, 2005). Feelings of disconnection arise when people feel unsupported and alienated, from themselves and others, and are demonstrated through a loss of voice. Voice is an indicator of self, and speaking one's feelings and thoughts is part of creating, maintaining and recreating one's authentic self (Jack, 1991: 32). When voice is diminished, for any reason, the outcome may be reduced support and understanding, when an *increased* need for support and understanding exists.

Evalyn demonstrated her loss of voice and sense that others didn't understand through being unable to speak about her concerns for her son; in particular, her concerns for his future well-being. Evalyn dealt with many challenges that her son's severe epilepsy and consequential intellectual disability had presented. She remained feeling isolated, especially with regard to her concerns for his future. A major concern for family carers is often the future welfare of their relative (Chambers, Ryan and Connor, 2001: 102). Evalyn described feeling different from other people; apart from them. She reported that colleagues, even when being compassionate, sympathetic or supportive, still didn't really understand:

Evalyn: [pause] I do feel different. People are very, I guess on the whole, people are pretty compassionate. They are very compassion-ate but I just don't think they really understand my life. And, I guess they don't have the same perspective on life as say, someone with a high support needs child has. Like, my child is nine years old now but, you know, for another parent with another nine-year-old child, they probably think, 'I've got another nine years where my child will live at home, stay at home'. But I, I don't know what the future is for my child, what will happen to him and ... that's something that really worries me about, you know, what will happen to Kevin. I obviously can't care for him forever ... So, you know, I'm always worried about the time when I can't look after him. And I don't think anyone ... really understands unless they've lived it or are living it. (Evalyn, Interview 1: 33; Vickers, 2005c: 211; Vickers and Parris, 2005: 97)

So, while Evalyn spoke of her colleagues being very compassionate, in the same breath she confirmed that they just didn't understand. One aspect of silencing the self that Jack highlighted involves women learning that the way to meet the needs of others is to deny the importance of their own needs and feelings, which subsequently inhibits their self-expression (Jack, 1991; DeMarco, Lynch and Board, 2002: 89). When Evalyn described her colleagues as compassionate, while concurrently acknowledging that they didn't understand her needs, feelings and concerns, she was diminishing and devaluing her self and her need to feel understood. Sometimes, women use a good deal of 'selective ignoring' of stressors which, unfortunately, tend to exacerbate rather than alleviate stress (Jena, 1999: 76). Unfortunately, she may also have been shutting off particular avenues of social and emotional support that may have assisted her in her own well-being (Vickers and Parris, 2005).

Dolly introduced the notion of being 'disconnected' from those around her. She spoke about her inability to network and socialise with the other mothers at the school that her daughter, Maggie, attended. I had thought she felt 'different' from the other mothers. Not quite:

Researcher: So you feel quite different from them [the other mothers]?

Dolly: Well, I feel a bit disconnected.

Researcher: Disconnected?

Dolly: Yes. Well, when I went to swimming it was great because I actually got to meet a couple of them ... but even things like, 'Can you stay and have lunch?' ... Well, I *couldn't*. But they all stayed and had lunch with each other. So, the couple of times I did that, it was lovely and then I felt bad because I wasn't working. So it was this constant guilt thing. (Dolly, Interview 1: 89–90; Vickers and Parris, 2005)

While there are no specific theoretical definitions of guilt, guilt seems to be associated with responsibility and action, whereas shame is more likely to be linked to self-image (Elvin-Nowak, 1999: 73). Conscious feelings of guilt are experienced by those whose actions (or inactions) are perceived to have injured another or have been contrary to the vital interests of another (Elvin-Nowak, 1999: 74). Dolly may have felt guilty when she wasn't at work; she wasn't being a 'good worker'. Concurrently, Dolly may have felt guilty for not spending enough time at her daughter's school; not being a 'good mother'. For Dolly to have felt guilt, a sense of responsibility was prerequisite. The ethic of care, teaching women what they 'should' be doing, would have 'assisted' enormously. Unfortunately, for many modern Western women, the illusion of choice about 'having it all' (Hewlett, 2002) serves to strengthen potential feelings of guilt. The individual woman is held accountable for how she uses her (illusory) modern freedom of choice while, in reality, many of the conditions she must abide by are already set by others' expectations. Women are expected to take responsibility for how childcare can be combined with work. When this breaks down – for any reason – it can lead to feelings of failure, followed by feelings of guilt (Elvin-Nowak, 1999: 76).

Dolly and others also confirmed their need for strong support networks and, sadly, their notable lack in this area. Dolly confirmed that she had no real network of support, other than her mother who she was currently not speaking to and who had recently been asked by Dolly to move out of the family home and discontinue her caring support role (Dolly, Interview 1: 36). Dolly had, for instance, no clue as to who was going to care for her child during the upcoming school holidays (the following week), when she had a full diary of work appointments scheduled (Dolly, Interview 1: 37).[1]

Researcher Note: *The issue of finding suitable carers is one that keeps coming up. In Dolly's case, she had, up until just before our first meeting, been relying very heavily on her mother to care for Maggie, especially in that window of time after school had finished, and before Dolly arrived home from work. However, one of the things that sparked a major argument between Dolly and her mother was Dolly's dissatisfaction with her mother's care of Maggie during that period. Dolly felt that her mother was* *not spending important time 'developing' Maggie; working with her, stimulating her, and playing with her in an active sense. Again, I find myself at something of a loss here, not being a mother and not really having a clue as to how I would have played with Maggie, where I would start looking for appropriate carers, or even a casual babysitter, having never had to think about it, let alone do it. However, I can certainly see how finding a carer you could trust with your child, especially a child with special needs, would not have been easy. What on earth would she do, especially at such short notice? I must ask her about this next time we meet.* (Vickers, Researcher Reflections, Wednesday, 16 April 2003)

This sense of disconnectedness, from colleagues, friends, partners, and other mothers, was shared by many of these women. During Stage 3, the Culminating Group Experience (CGE), both Wendy and Evalyn confirmed the magnitude of this issue for them. Wendy said:

Wendy: Yes ... I was really looking forward to being able to talk with other people about the experiences and how they managed things. When Margaret said there was that third phase, I thought, 'Oh good', because I don't really talk to anybody else. There isn't an association that embraces our situation. So I thought it would be really good to just talk with other people about what their experience was. (Wendy, CGE: 8)

Dolly specifically reported feeling 'disconnected' from those around her and had raised the issue of not being able to team up with other mothers of children with disabilities for support because of her heavy work schedule. Dolly owned (in conjunction with her ex-husband) a human resources consultancy firm, requiring her to work long hours. Indeed, working full-time was the major factor that set her apart from the other mothers at her daughter's school:

Dolly: A lot of the mothers don't work. They're on pensions or maintenance or whatever else. So it's, without seeming precious, they're not corporate women. They're sort of more *'mums'* that might have two or three other children, and they've had a Down's [child with Down's syndrome] or they've had a child with a disability. And they're either married and their husband's supporting them to be at home to look after the other children and so they can spend time down at the school, or they're single mums who are living on maintenance and pensions and are able, again, to be more flexible in terms of what they do during the day as well. I mean, I'm sure some of them work but most of them seem to have lots of flexibility. (Dolly, Interview 1: 88; Vickers, 2005b)

Dolly's sense of disconnection stemmed directly from her inability to be with others living in a similar situation; to share with them, to rely on them, to have the flexibility that they apparently had with their caring responsibilities. One possible explanation for the reported sense of 'otherness' that the women in this study felt may well be directly related to the limited opportunities they had to interact with others who *would* understand. Several others mentioned that they were also unable to socialise with other mothers of children with chronic illness.

Dolly's reported feelings of guilt also included: guilt about her 'lesser' contributions to school activities; guilt about time spent away from work; and, guilt that she was not there with her child. This guilt is 'everyday guilt'; guilt that is always more or less present and that is brought to the fore and accentuated under certain conditions (Elvin-Nowak, 1999: 77) – such as a researcher asking about it. These guilt feelings are often expressed in other ways: insufficiency, dissatisfaction, burden, and 'shoulds' (Elvin-Nowak, 1999: 77). Dolly may also have felt guilt because of her limited capacity for time-consuming engagement in her daughter's school activities. The modern illusion of choice for women contributes to them being blamed by others if they make the 'wrong' choices:

Dolly: I feel really bad ... Maggie's got an Easter hat thing today, and I can't be there for it. So I spent hours with super-glue, completely ruined the counter out the front, with feathers and all that sort of stuff. And, you know, it would be really nice to go. I went to the swimming carnival last week, but could only stay for an hour, or half an hour ... But you do feel, I do feel almost discriminated against ... And last year I was able to go swimming, taking Maggie swimming ... So I volunteered and Steven [Dolly's ex-husband and now business partner] was being really supportive of this, of me going down and spending an hour. But, you know, it took probably more like two and a half by the time you drive down, you walk the kids from the classroom to the pool, you change them, you swim with them for half an hour, and then you get them dressed, and then you take them back to the classroom. It's a couple of hours and then you come home. And then you have a shower and get dressed and come to work, so probably more like three hours lost all up in that exercise, which is almost half a day's work but, you know [slight sigh], I got a little award saying, 'Thank you for your participation' ... Certainly, the school and the principal, they just generally favour more involvement. They really actively encourage you to be really involved, which would be really nice to be. But then there's that trade-off. You know, like I can't afford to feed her if I can't work, you know.

Researcher: Do you think they, do you get a sense that they appreciate, for you, the enormity of taking half a day out of your working week?

Dolly: No, I don't think they do. No. No. (Dolly, Interview 1: 87–88; Vickers and Parris, 2005: 98)

The question of guilt that mothers felt, raised earlier, is an important one. Elements of shame are linked to shortcomings in one's personal traits ('I am a bad mother') which, in turn, generate feelings of guilt (Elvin-Nowak, 1999: 77). This guilt is associated with the existence of a relationship. The guilt situation emerges when the guilt object (for example, Dolly's daughter) is seen as completely without responsibility. They are 'injured' by the 'bad behaviour' of the guilty person. However, Dolly's sense of guilt is not associated with any *actual* injured party. Maggie is fine. The ethic of care, described in Chapter 1, promotes women's ideas of injured parties (like children) that result from the behaviour of the 'bad mother'. The ethic of care and the associated 'shoulds' also support women silencing themselves.

In Jack's (1991) study, women also thought that silencing themselves was what they *should* do, and that any sense of alienation they felt was also, somehow, their own fault. However, Dolly gave no indication that this was what she believed – quite the reverse. She wanted understanding and acknowledgement that her caring responsibilities were hard work, and not easily managed. Professional carers have noted, for example, that caring work is extremely difficult, involving physical and emotional labour, and very stressful (Jenkins, 2004). However, Jenkins also reinforces the fact that such work is often understated and diminished. Women are often sought to work with children, for example, because they are viewed as cheap and flexible (Jenkins, 2004). Dolly's efforts at the local school were similarly unappreciated. Ironically, Dolly's time was anything but cheap and flexible, despite expectations to the contrary.

Cate's sense of 'otherness' was magnified by the response of her colleagues to her son's autism. Cate's colleagues unwittingly aided in ensuring her silence and, at the same time, further limited her access to important emotional, psychological and social support. There was evidence of stigma being ascribed to Cate's son, William. Autism is certainly an illness that would attract 'social-discomfort stigma', especially as it related to behavioural deviations (Vickers, 2000: 143). The social discomfort became apparent via the changes evident in Cate's relationships with her colleagues as the news emerged that her child had autism. Cate initially spoke of how she used to relate with her colleagues – *before* the diagnosis of her son's illness:

> **Cate:** What happened was, when you're at work and you're pregnant, it's a big deal. People know; they can see it. And it's, 'Wow, a kid's going to be born'. And then when they're born, everyone's asking you about the kid and what they are doing. And you develop relationships with other people who have kids of the same age. So then come the comparisons and the milestones that they reach when they're doing that. And a couple of people here have kids of the same age, and what happened was I would be, 'No. He didn't talk yet'. 'Well, my daughter says "shoe" now'. And I would say, 'Well, mine doesn't say anything. And all he does is go like this [indicates the child's movements] all day'. (Cate, Interview 1: 7; Vickers and Parris, 2005: 99)

Prior to being silenced and disconnected, Cate *had been* talking about her son's unusual behaviour and slower-than-usual development. However, once her son was diagnosed with autism, things changed. Cate's colleagues no longer asked about her child, giving her no opportunity to discuss her son's difficulties, how she felt about them or, importantly, what she needed – effectively silencing her and disconnecting her from access to possible avenues of support. She admitted to changes in her relationships at work:

> **Researcher:** Do you feel different or misunderstood by colleagues, or excluded or alienated in any way because of William?
> **Cate:** Just from the ones that I was friendlier with about the kids. Just those guys. They're really nice to me every day. They're never mean to me, ever. But we just kind of don't talk like we used to. And it's kind of like, 'Oh well. Now Cate's one of *them*. She's not one of *us* anymore'. But that's, you know, that's OK [voice slightly dropped]. (Cate Interview 1: 12; Vickers and Parris, 2005: 99)

The drop in Cate's voice suggested that, from her point of view, her colleagues' behaviour was not OK and that she was feeling hurt and rejected, even while outwardly stating that their behaviour was acceptable. She was, to some extent, silencing her grief response here, by making assurances that her colleagues' behaviour was OK with her, when clearly it was not. Cate also highlighted her experience of 'us' and 'them':

> **Researcher Note:** *The comment about Cate being one of 'them' leapt out at me. As a person with a highly stigmatised, disabling chronic illness, I could relate to what she might have been thinking when speaking of being relegated to being one of 'them'. Ironically, Cate's work organisation is one that offers support to people with disabilities in the community. I am assuming that the other workers in Cate's workplace unconsciously differentiate between the clients (those with disabilities – 'them') and the staff (those without disabilities – 'us'). I have had numerous experiences with other people's discomfort with my disability. People often have difficulty speaking about it. For example, few will ask me directly about having MS. They will ask, instead, about: my 'health'; my 'problems'; my 'condition'; how I am 'in myself'. While I look pretty normal at the moment, I did have to use a walking stick for a period of about 18 months. This proved extremely discomforting for many: they stared; they looked when they thought I wasn't looking; they looked the other way (very obviously); they pretended the walking stick didn't exist; they scoffed, thinking that a 'young' person like me didn't need it. I was experiencing the stigma of physical disability. So, when Cate said that her colleagues thought 'she's not one of "us" anymore',* I got it. (Vickers, Researcher Reflections, Thursday, 17 July 2003)

The obtrusiveness of the stigma (Goffman, 1963; Nettleton, 1995: 91; Vickers, 2000: 143) ascribed to Cate's son resulted in Cate being silenced by her colleagues. The social discomfort that Cate's colleagues experienced because of William's autism were, ultimately, contributing to the stigmatisation that Cate experienced, as well as in Cate inhibiting her self-expression and action to avoid conflict and the possible loss of the relationship (DeMarco, Lynch and Board, 2002: 90) with her friends at work. Like the women in Jack's (1991) study, Cate may well have been silencing herself to avoid giving her colleagues a reason to reject her (Jack, 1991: 138). However, unlike the women in Jack's study, Cate's colleagues contributed to her silence. The outcome for Cate was reduced emotional support as she struggled to balance the demands of her multiple roles and caring responsibilities (Vickers and Parris, 2005) and deal with her ongoing and unacknowledged grief (discussed further in Chapter 4).

Doing it all

What also repeatedly arose in the stories was these women's overwhelming sense of having to 'do it all'; of always having to respond, take responsibility, plan, consider, worry – and with the very definite sense that those around them rarely understood their continuing, multiple and, often, conflicting and exhausting responsibilities. Where male partners were present, even in positive relationships, the women commented that it was always the school who called *them* first (not their partner); that *they* were the ones who took their child to the doctor, or to counseling, or to whatever professional consultation was required. Mothers working outside the home are usually the ones to take the child to the required medical and professional appointments, and to stay with the child during hospitalisations (Gibson, 1995: 1205). This was confirmed by the women in this study; others merely 'help' with 'her job' (Burke et al, 1999; Vickers, Parris and Bailey, 2004). Sadly, in the majority of cases, male partners were absent – physically, emotionally, or financially.

All respondents reported, in some form or another, a feeling of being expected to do more than their share – to 'do it all'. Many of them also commented about this in specific relation to the role and contribution of their partner (or ex-partner). They felt that they shouldered the lion's share of responsibility for their child's well-being, being continually the ones to ensure caring responsibilities were not left to chance. Even when supportive relationships were evident (and, mostly, they were not), these women reported that they were ultimately responsible for the child's welfare and development, and for all decisions and actions surrounding that (Vickers and Parris, 2005).

Dolly reported the lack of pragmatic, physical assistance from her ex-husband. In Chapter 2, Dolly lamented that she was always the one to buy Maggie's medication; organise the doctor's appointments; take her child for blood tests; wash the clothes; iron the clothes; buy the clothes; change the bed; organise the nappies; do the grocery shopping; and, get Maggie's shoes fitted. You will also recall Dolly's anger when the perfect little overnight bag, packed for her daughter's weekends with her father, came back full of dirty washing (Dolly, Interview 1: 90; Vickers, Parris and Bailey, 2004; Vickers and Parris, 2005). Dolly described how difficult it was when she had been sick with the flu – and still had to do it all:

> **Dolly:** The reality is Maggie *does* need, and *I* need, a full-time helper in my life, and her life ... Like last week, I actually had this flu thing, and I felt quite awful on the Tuesday. Well, you know, too bad. You know, *too bad!* I had to get up. The last thing I wanted to do was get out of bed. Had to get up, get Maggie organised. And Steven wouldn't dream of thinking to come over and help out or change an appointment or anything like that ... Shelley's [Dolly's mother] always been there. Now she's moved out, I don't think he really understands all the additional load now that I do, because I could say to Shelley, 'Look, here's Maggie's script. Can you take that up?' But now I have to do all that as well. (Dolly, Interview 1: 37–38)

Sandra also talked a great deal about her experience of doing it all. She reported (Interview 1: 1), having taken her son, Edward, with her everywhere when he was a baby with serious and chronic tonsillitis – even to work. She described 'having him on her hip' as she went about her business day and a 'baby gurgling in the background' during meetings with clients. For Sandra, doing it all meant bringing in the money, managing the household, and keeping the family together emotionally. As her son got older and became plagued with problems-related to ADD, Sandra reported that it was still always *she* who received the calls from the school if there was a problem; that it was *she* who went to school evenings and spoke with the teachers; that it was *she* who organised the doctor's visits and counseling that were required. She felt very resentful about this and believed that it added immeasurably to the strain of an already difficult situation. She also admitted that she was unhappy that her partner, Robert, was not able to provide more emotional support when it was needed (Sandra, Interview 1: 9).

Spousal support has been noted as being most important for mothers of children with chronic illness (Ray, 2002: 431). Sadly, of the nine women who participated in this study, just three reported supportive partner relationships (Polly, Sally, and Evalyn), although the primary responsibility for responding to the needs of their child still remained with them. Dolly, Oitk, Wendy, and Charlene reported being separated or divorced from their partners, and both Sandra and Cate demonstrated that their partners, while still present in the relationship, were less than supportive; in some situations, adding significantly to their burden. Fathers tend not to have the same investment in caring responsibilities for a child and, as a result, their confidence and expertise in relation to the chronic illness or disability is not developed over time, and certainly not commensurately with the mother's (Gibson, 1995: 1205) which may explain some of this reticence.

> **Researcher Note:** *However, I do not assume that all fathers fall into this category. Bianchi (2000) has reported that there is mounting evidence to suggest that married fathers, in particular, have significantly increased the time they are spending with children (in late 1990s compared to around 1965). Thus, it may be that fathers are also increasingly facing this problem, especially as responsibility for child caring shifts over time and fathers are increasingly prepared to take on such responsibilities.* (Vickers, Researcher Reflections, Friday, 15 August 2003)

However, it wasn't just that male partners were less competent and helpful, or lower in confidence and expertise. In some cases, they were seen to actively make matters worse – sometimes significantly worse. Cate described such a situation where her husband actually created a hindrance to her caring work:

> **Cate:** And another place that's really hard is when you go shopping at the supermarket. There are tons of things that set him [William] off. And ... there's just a certain way you have to do it, and that's the only way it can be done. It's done by careful research by me; therefore Colin [Cate's partner] *never* goes, because if he goes, he'll just mess up my system. *And he makes fun of me* anyway, because I have a certain way. I'm like, 'Colin, you can't do it *that* way because it won't work.' There's food items that set him off; there's sights that set him off. (Cate, Interview 1: 24; emphasis added)

Cate was silencing herself here in two ways: 'dividing herself' (presenting an outer compliant self while experiencing inner hostility) (Jack, 1991: 169) and 'externalising herself' (basing her behaviour on the rules constructed by the social group) (DeMarco, Lynch and Board, 2002: 90; Vickers and Parris, 2005). Cate reported doing the shopping – with her autistic son present, and her husband absent – because it was easier for her than being *mocked* by her husband, arguing with him, upsetting her routine with her son, and transforming a mundane task into a nightmare (Vickers and Parris, 2005). Notably, Cate also appeared to have done the shopping because it was 'her job'. She fitted in the shopping, caring, cooking and other home duties, around caring for her four-year-old with autism, her full-time job, raising her other dependent two-year-old, and caring for her adult brother with a disability who also lived in the household. However, at no time did Cate suggest that it *should* be this way, that caring about her needs was selfish, or that ignoring her needs was morally right (Jack, 1991: 155).

Cate also reported difficulties communicating with her partner and eliciting his support. She confessed that they had never discussed their child's condition. Cate appeared to be using the psychological defence of repression to respond to her fears in this area (Oldham and Kleiner, 1990):

> **Cate:** We don't really talk a lot about William. I'm still observing him. This opens up a lot of areas for me personally, because my father did not accept my brother. It was a huge, *huge* thing in our house ... He [Cate's father] was really, really not into my brother. He was abusive in the home. It was really hard. Really, really hard. I spent a lot of time protecting my brother from him, in all kinds of ways. And taking the brunt of stuff for him in all kinds of ways. I guess on some level I thought that my husband would have the same reaction ... But that's why I don't really talk about it, because I don't want to go there.
> **Researcher:** You're frightened something might come out that you don't want?
> **Cate:** Yes, I don't want to hear [Colin] say he thinks it's my fault or he thinks that he [William] is whatever; and pick a negative thing ... If I had trouble, they'd be on a plane like that [snaps her fingers to indicate an immediate response]. They'd come up here right away. But I'm not sure how ... these guys are not equipped to watch him [William] every day ... He's just too bizarre for them. (Cate, Interview 1: 15–16)

Note the apparent contradiction in Cate's assertions: On the one hand, she states that her parents-in-law would drop everything to help her if she needed it. On the other hand, she admits that her son's autistic behaviour was just 'too bizarre' for them to care for him on a long-term or regular basis. These kinds of contradictions point to her likely levels of stress, conflict and ambivalence. Sandra, like Cate, also experienced communication difficulties with her partner. Sandra felt that her partner was not coping well with their son's problems with ADD. I asked her about this during the second interview:

Researcher: You also noted that Robert didn't cope really well with the fact that Edward had something wrong with him – this is in the early stages – that he appeared to ... deny it. Can you tell me exactly, perhaps give me an example, what you mean when you say that Robert didn't cope very well?

Sandra: He just would try, he would know that something was wrong with him but he wouldn't acknowledge there was something wrong with him.

Researcher: So, if you spoke about it, what would happen?

Sandra: He just doesn't want to know; he'd just change the subject. Interestingly, Edward's report at the end of last term was atrocious, and it arrived in the holidays. Robert just said to him, 'I'm not happy. We will discuss this on the day before you go back to school, so that you can set objectives'. And the day before Edward went back to school, I said to him, 'We need to talk to Edward about this', and he went, 'No. He knows I'm not happy'. (Sandra, Interview 2: 7)

Sandra's frustration with her partner was evident. She wanted *both* of them to discuss the report card with their son before he returned to school. However, Robert's response – to do nothing – must have been very disheartening and frustrating. Robert appeared to be denying or repressing his son's problems at school, a defence mechanism (Oldham and Kleiner, 1990) reinforced by his apparent inability or lack of desire to deal with the issues of concern. Sandra related another incident where she and Robert were speaking to a friend about Edward and that, 'Robert just walked away. He couldn't deal with it' (Sandra, Interview 1: 9). For Sandra, while Robert did not actively work against her, his actions resulted in Sandra almost having another 'child' to care for and be responsible for – in a life already overwhelmed with caring responsibility. What Sandra needed was reliable, adult support. Sandra gave another example where her partner, Robert, could not be the adult in this relationship:

Sandra: We knew that giving Edward coloured drinks sent him [Edward] off the wall. We went somewhere in two cars, and Robert stopped at a garage and brought him red drink and Twisties and everything. And we got out of the car and he was hanging off the ceiling [sound of incredulity]. To support that, you know, 'No mate, you know that's not good for you. Let's go for the things that are OK'.

Researcher: Do you think that Robert did that because he just wasn't really aware because he hadn't been at the consultations with you?
Sandra: He *knew*, but it was like he wouldn't deny his son what he wanted. (Sandra, Interview 2: 9)

Cate, Dolly, Sally and Sandra all discussed frankly their difficulties in actually talking to their partners about the problems that their children experienced, and the impact that this had on them, individually and collectively, as a couple and as a family. As part of the action research agenda, I asked Sandra what she would have liked her partner to have done differently:

Sandra: With Edward, to be consistent in his involvement with him. Because there's been these extremes of, 'You are my perfect son and I've given you 150 per cent of my attention. You and I are like that'. [Sandra indicates their closeness with her fingers entwined]. And then he'll drop him because he's so focused on something else that's work-related and doesn't give him time. So, I would have liked him to have been more consistent. I would have liked him to have been involved in taking him to the doctor's, taking him to the specialist. He's been to the specialist's twice in all of these years. He needs to –, it's almost like acknowledging to Edward that there is an issue and we're working together. (Sandra, Interview 2: 9)

Sandra did not want to be doing it all, but wanted to be working together with Robert in dealing with Edward. For Cate, where support in home duties was also lacking, she felt unable to leave her disabled child with his own father for any length of time. You will recall (see Chapter 2), that Cate came home from work early to find both her autistic four-year-old and his two-year-old sister home alone – their father had gone out to buy himself more alcohol. Cate's response? To manufacture a schedule so her husband was never left at home alone with their son, a requirement that would be difficult for most parents to achieve, but especially difficult for Cate who had little familial caring support at hand. It also reinforced her experience of doing it all:

Cate: I don't know. We never talk about it. I never sat down and said, 'I don't trust you'. I just kind of manufacture our schedule so that it doesn't occur. But the closest I ever came was, 'If you feel like you're going to flip out, you've got to call me. That's the rule'. (Cate, Interview 1: 63)

Cate was understandably furious with Colin for leaving the two children home alone. However, it is possible that, at some level, she also experienced some guilt as a result of 'allowing' this to happen – not being a 'good mother'. Cate may also have been furious that she had to continue with the constant burden of caring for her children, with so little support, and unable to find a way out of her situation (Elvin-Nowak, 1999: 79). Being unable to rely on her partner with regard to such an essential aspect of the caring process may well have fuelled her anger, ambivalence, and possibly, feelings of guilt.

While not always as vivid and disconcerting as Cate's experiences, lack of partner support was *frequently* reported. Levels of support from partners varied wildly and many made it very clear that stronger, more proactive support from the partner would have been most welcome. Anger and frustration were frequently reported towards partners who were emotionally absent, or unhelpful in a pragmatic sense, or both. It is noted that not all partners are capable of providing the emotional support needed for such a difficult situation (McGrath, 2001: 200). However, Sandra rallied against the pressure to silence herself on this issue, feeling resentful. Her learning was demonstrated as she reported a change in her response to such situations:

Researcher: I want to ask you about *you* now ... What, for you, would be an escape?
Sandra: Somebody to take it off me for a while.
Researcher: To take it off you, so you don't have to think about any of it and worry?
Sandra: [Nodding] I think too, I've got better at [it]. I had some major appointments I had to be at on Tuesday and Wednesday and, when Robert's mother rang me on Tuesday morning to say that Dad wasn't well and could I come and get her and take her to the hospital, I just cancelled [the scheduled appointments]. I didn't participate. I let other people do it and I didn't worry about it. I think I'm getting better. It mightn't happen the same way as if I'm there [at work], but that's OK. And if we lose business, we lose business. Really, at the end of the day, I can only do what I can do ... Yes. Look, I think I probably take on too much at times. I should just say to Robert, 'I'm too busy. I've got my work things'. (Sandra, Interview 2: 14–15; Vickers and Parris, 2005: 103)

For many women, the rules constructed by the social group are not necessarily congruent with what she values (DeMarco, Lynch and Board, 2002: 90), but she will follow them anyway. However, in Sandra's case, she did her best to work around them. She refused, for instance, to 'externalise herself' (DeMarco, Lynch and Board, 2002: 90). When her son was just a few months old and very sick, and she was running her own business, she did not 'self-sacrifice' herself (DeMarco, Lynch and Board, 2002: 90) or her career by giving up work to look after her baby. Instead, Sandra broke traditional social conventions by bringing her child to the office to care for him – although it is noted that it was still *she* who had to do this (Vickers and Parris, 2005). Sally's exasperation with her partner also emerged during the interviews. At first she portrayed her partner, Peter, as very easy-going. However, she signaled her frustration as the interview progressed. Phrases like 'it's all too hard' said it all:

> **Sally:** Sometimes I just think it's all too hard; it's just in the too-hard basket; I don't want to do it anymore. And sometimes too, I can remember, there's been times when I've had battles with trying to get good health services for her or good educational support for her, and you get so emotionally caught up in those kind of battles just to make sure that she gets a fair *go*, that it all just becomes really hard and just really draining. I tend to be the one that takes that stuff on, because Peter's fairly easy-going. So it tends to be with me, otherwise it won't happen. (Sally, Interview 1: 7; Vickers and Parris, 2005: 102)

Sally made it clear that she shouldn't have to always be the one to battle with professionals to ensure her daughter's care. Certainly, it has been noted in the literature that the dealings of mothers with professionals are often highly problematic as they try to get care for their child. Encounters are frequently based on conflict, and the mother's worth and character are continually scrutinised (Todd and Jones, 2003: 229). Sally's psychological, physical and emotional fatigue indicated she was fed up with handling all the battles alone.

Clearly, the question of partner support is a big one (beyond the scope of this chapter). However, it is raised here to highlight the magnitude of the weight of responsibility that these women carried. Unfortunately, many carers of children with chronic illness have come to the conclusion that they are alone in the responsibility of caring, and that this made the challenge all the more difficult (Ray, 2002:

434). Seeking and accepting help is a vital constituent to positive coping and making their 'invisible' work visible to others: learning what is needed, getting beyond others' discomfort and lack of understanding, and being specific about the help that is needed, is recommended for parents of children with chronic illness (Ray, 2002: 434).

Actionable knowledge commences

An important component of action research is the development of actionable knowledge, learning what things can make life better. I conclude this chapter with other examples of how this actionable knowledge was developing. During the second interview, Sandra spoke about her need to 'pass back' some of the burden of responsibility for family caring:

> **Researcher:** If you had your time over, would you respond to the situation with Robert [Sandra's partner] differently?
> **Sandra:** Differently [nodding].
> **Researcher:** Yes, what would you do?
> **Sandra:** ... I wouldn't take on the carer role for him to the level that I've been the protector for him for such a long-time. And I did it initially out of huge love and trying to make it better and help him, and all I did was really just give him more and more reason not to be involved.
> **Researcher:** Allowed him to *not* take responsibility?
> **Sandra:** Yes, yes. ... And I've often thought to myself that I've created a rod for myself, because I have; I've taken everything on. (Sandra, Interview 2: 7)

Learning is evident in Sandra's behaviour. Other respondents also indicated changes in their behaviour. For example, Polly started showing concern for herself by walking to lose weight and get fit, while Oitk made the necessary changes to her work schedule to continue her psychology degree, a vital constituent in her life. Wendy also started drawing more on her ex-husband for pragmatic support.

What was evident here was the meaningful connection between reflection and action by the women in this study. Sandra's comments confirmed that actionable knowledge was being accumulated and reflected upon. Action researchers confirm that the only meaningful way to theorise is through successive cycles of combined reflection and action, the action feeding back to revise the reflection in ongoing cycles (Greenwood, 2002: 125). Here, participants were reflecting on their circumstances, behaviour, and feelings, and responding to that. As Greenwood (2002: 127) confirms, action research is not about imposing expert knowledge on stakeholders, but is about the sharing of knowledge – often very different – between researchers and participants in a manner that is helpful and can ameliorate problems. There was evidence that this was commencing – and I was delighted.

4
Unacknowledged Grief

He Never Did

My son, he is four, he has autism
He doesn't speak; different sounds, not words
His own language, alien language
I understand it.

His first experience with daycare, you'd think he would cry
He never did
He licked the wall, flapping his hands
He touches things, puts them in his mouth, looked at everything.

He didn't even know when I came to pick him up
Did he recognise me?
I couldn't tell. I can't tell. I'm not sure
It took him a while to even come over to me – I'd go to him.

After a few weeks he started to recognise me
I think he knew who I was
But he wouldn't come to me like, 'It's mum!'
No. He never did.

(Cate, Interview 1: 1–2)

The data poem above, created from Cate's words, is a poignant reminder of one possible area of ongoing grief in Cate's life that others may not be aware of: the grief surrounding her desire for her son to know and love and recognise her. This chapter begins by talking about grief and the need to acknowledge that grief exists in people's lives and in organisations; that 'there is always grief in the room', be it experienced by one who has lost a close family member, been diagnosed

81

with a serious illness, or who has lost their job. The grief that these women experienced existed for them, both at home and at work, and involved characteristics generally not included in traditional models of grief, such as ongoing, recurring and multiple sources of grief. Unlike the grief associated with a death in the family, their grief was chronic and tied inexorably to the health of their child. Their grief also emanated from multiple sources, for example: losses experienced by their child as a result of illness or disability; changes and losses in their own lives; lost or changed relationships; and lost income or career opportunities. Finally, the grief they experienced could emerge at any time; daily events, large or small, could act as triggers. From the hospitalisation of their child, through to the thoughtless comment of a colleague; the grief they experienced was lived at work and at home.

The first section explores the literature on grief and its potential limitations. I then share narratives that depict three themes of grief:

- Grief from a life changing event;
- Ongoing and recurring grief; and,
- Multiple sources of grief.

'There's always grief in the room': bounded grief at work

As a colleague of ours once remarked, there is always grief some-where in the room. One person may be feeling personal pain due to a death in the family. Another may find personality conflicts in the workplace unbearable. Still another may be watching a colleague struggle with a serious illness and not know how to help. (Dutton et al, 2002: 6)

Grief is a painful and, unfortunately, common experience (Bonanno and Kaltman, 2001: 705). However, the idea that grief exists in our workplaces is rarely recognised. The question of how grief adversely affects workplace performance is also rarely considered (Eyetsemitan, 1998: 469). Conservative estimations of the cost of grief to organisa-tions is in the billions of dollars (Bolyard, 1983; Myers, 1984; McClelland, 1985; Eyetsemitan, 1998: 470). Unfortunately, a lack of understanding of the grieving process, false assumptions about emo-tional attachments that result in grief (Eyetsemitan, 1998: 474), plus a lack of acknowledgement of all the possible sources of grief that may affect us – both from home and work – all combine to limit or bind the understanding of grief experienced in our life and work (Vickers, 2005c).

Grief and bereavement are usually only associated with death. Most of us would recognise grief as deep or intense sorrow; something that can cause keen distress or suffering (Wilkes, 1979: 643; Vickers, 2005c). Similarly, to bereave is to deprive someone of something or someone valued, especially through death (Wilkes, 1979: 137; Vickers, 2005c). However, there is much more to know about grief. There are numerous descriptors of grief: normal and abnormal grief; pathological grief; complicated grief; unresolved or chronic grief; inhibited grief; delayed grief; absent grief; denied grief; a prolonged absence of grief; exaggerated grief; masked grief; chronic mourning; distorted mourning; and inhibited mourning (Bonanno and Kaltman, 2001: 707–709; Noppe, 2000; Vickers 2005c). I wish to vivify the absence of understanding and recognition of grief as it was experienced by these women, at work and at home, and the likely outcome of their grief being bound, hidden or constrained, especially grief that didn't fall into traditional categories and follow traditionally assumed trajectories.

The literature on grief includes discussions of the tasks of grieving (Worden, 1991; Eyetsemitan, 1998; Noppe, 2000); grieving work (Stroebe and Stroebe, 1991); phases of grieving to be endured (Kubler-Ross, 1969); and whether bereavement characteristics are universally observed or tempered by a myriad of individual differences such as culture, gender, developmental level or personality (Noppe, 2000: 520). The manifestations of grief vary widely. On one hand, there may be positive outcomes: positive thoughts, beliefs and appraisals – and laughter (Bonanno and Kaltman, 2001). However, more frequently noted grief reactions include mental lapses, decreased energy, difficulty in making decisions, anxiety, helplessness, an inability to concentrate, preoccupation, social withdrawal, and weeping (Eyetsemitan, 1998: 469; Vickers, 2005c). Also: cognitive disorganisation; confusion and preoccupation; disturbance of identity; a disrupted sense of future; a long-term search for meaning; dysphoria; pining or yearning; loneliness; negative health effects; mortality; disrupted social functioning and isolation; role disruptions; and difficulties with new relationships (Bonanno and Kaltman, 2001; Vickers, 2005c). Scholars of organisations, gender, families and health all need to be concerned about grief.

Grief and bereavement can be experienced as a result of life events other than death. Certainly, the most typical and recognised source of grief is the death of a close family member or partner (Eyetsemitan, 1998). Models of mourning and grieving bolster this assumption. For example, Worden's (1991) four tasks of mourning urge the bereaved to: (1) accept the reality of the loss; (2) work through the pain of grief; (3) adjust to the environment in which the deceased is missing; and (4) emotionally relocate the deceased and move on with life (Eyetsemitan, 1998: 473). However, models like these take little account of chronic or ongoing grief, and grief that reemerges and reasserts itself despite frequent urging to the bereaved to 'move on'. Such models fail to recognise grief that might be multiple-sourced, or that spills from home into the workday. For example: grief associated with the onset or exacerbation of a significant chronic illness (Vickers, 2001a); the impending death of a loved one (Krohn, 1998); contradictory emotions of grief, joy, hope and fear, for mothers of children with significant developmental disabilities (Larson, 1998: 865); or grief associated with undergoing fertility treatment (Lukse and Vacc, 1999) – all offer possible scenarios where grief might be taken to work. Similarly, numerous sources of grief can emanate – unrecognised – from the workplace and spill over to home. I have elsewhere (Vickers, 2005c) described the grief surrounding toxic workplaces and toxic emotions at work (Frost, 2003); emotionally anorexic workplaces (Fineman, 1993a; 1993b); redundancies and downsizing (Kets de Vries and Balazs, 1997; Stein, 1998; 2001; Vickers, 2002b); bullying and violence at work (Rees, 1995; Mann, 1996; Randall, 1997; Vickers, 2001c; Barron, 2002); alienating workplaces (Blauner, 1964; Fromm, 1963/1994; La Bier, 1986; Braverman, 1994); and abusive workplaces (Powell, 1998; Perrone and Vickers, 2004; Vickers, 2004). Finally, disenfranchised grief requires recognition of losses that are not socially sanctioned, for example: extramarital affairs; homosexual relationships; bereavement based on relationships with deceased that are not based on recognisable kin ties (eg lovers, friends, neighbours, colleagues); or past relationships (eg ex-spouses, past lovers or former friends) (Eyetsemitan, 1998: 470–471; Vickers, 2005c).

Even with traditional models of grief, the tendency is still to underestimate the effects of loss, and to underestimate how intensely distressing and disabling loss is, and how long the distress may last (Bowlby, 1980: 8; Eyetsemitan, 1998). It is supposed that a normal healthy person can and should get over recognised grief fairly rapidly and completely (Bowlby, 1980: 8). However, grief is experienced differently, by different people (Bonanno and Kaltman, 2001: 705), and should not be viewed as a uniform process. Rather, it is a course determined by a variety of factors, such as gender, cultural context, and the age of survivors (Noppe, 2000: 533). There are also marked individual differences in the intensity and duration of grief. Some grieve openly and deeply for a year, only slowly returning to a semblance of normal functioning over time. Others suffer intensely, but for a shorter period (Vickers, 2005c). Others appear to get over their losses almost immediately and to move on with sufficient ease as to raise doubts in others about their hiding something or running away from their pain (Bonanno and Kaltman, 2001: 705–706). There remains little agreement about what might constitute normal grief, when grief might be considered abnormal, nor what might be its routine manifestations (Noppe, 2000: 520). Flawed assumptions and faulty knowledge about grief combine poorly with expectations about workplace behaviour, to the detriment of the grieving individual. The result can be 'stifled grief', grief denied its full course of mourning (Eyetsemitan, 1998: 470), or 'bounded grief', grief that is not enabled, and not freely lived, recognised, acknowledged or understood (Vickers, 2005c).

There remains little recognition of the experience of grief – at work and at home. Tension exists, in particular, between grief reactions and work; expressions of the urge to weep, or appeals to others for help, inevitably carry with them an admission of weakness (Bowlby, 1980: 27). Grieving behaviours such as those listed above are generally deemed to be inappropriate workplace behaviour (Eyetsemitan, 1998: 469). The grieving rules that exist in our communities and organisations tend to specify very narrowly who, when, where, how, for how long, and for which people, we are allowed to grieve (Eyetsemitan, 1998: 469). In the workplace especially, enabling exemptions from normal responsibilities because of grief, as well as the receipt of social and emotional support, tends to follow normalised rules of grieving. Personnel policies codify society's grief rules (Eyetsemitan, 1998: 471) and while these policies may vary with, for example, parental or spousal loss being presumed greater than the loss of a friend (Eyetsemitan, 1998: 476), the grieving period is still formally (and narrowly) determined. Even for 'recognised' grief events, the few days leave allocated to 'recover' from the death of a spouse or child will be insufficient to enable grief to be experienced over its full course (Vickers, 2005c). As Dutton and colleagues remind us, you cannot 'ask people to check their emotions at the door' (Dutton et al, 2002: 61). Sadly, in organisations especially, this is often what is expected.

At a time when claims are being made that work is becoming more central to our lives and identities (Trinca and Fox, 2004), support for workers should be paramount. Recognising grief, at work and crossing over between home and work, are important steps forward. Working in times of trauma requires the case for compassion to be made (Dutton et al, 2002). Even traditional sources of grief and their manifestation at work deserves more thought, with 97 per cent of people reporting having been bereaved at least once while working; and 47 per cent more than once (Eyetsemitan, 1998: 475). Of these, 84 per cent reported resuming full-blown responsibilities immediately after returning to work, with 64 per cent receiving no further support, and only 14 per cent receiving informal support from coworkers. Suggestions made to employers by those bereaved included: (a) to offer more time off work and/or show support (37 per cent); (b) to provide counseling or professional help (29 per cent); and (c) to show concern and understanding (27 per cent). Of interest and despite assumptions to the contrary, *work was mentioned just 0.04 per cent of the time* as a way the organisation could help their employees cope with bereavement (Eyetsemitan, 1998: 475).

Narratives of grief

There has been an important shift in the last two decades away from the stereotypical portrayal of children with disabilities as being a 'problem', and their mother as a 'tragedy-stricken' individual (Redmond and Richardson, 2003: 205). Having a child with special needs is no longer considered primarily a story of gloom and doom (Barnett et al, 2003: 185). Nevertheless, it is vital that the grief these mothers experience be acknowledged – at work and at home. Parental reactions to the diagnosis of a chronic illness are determined by a complex set of processes related to personality, relationship history and how one has learned to process information about emotions and relationships. The process by which parents come to terms with their reactions is not yet fully understood (Barnett et al, 2003: 187). However, we do know that parenting a child with a chronic condition is an emotional experience (Johnston and Marder, 1994).

The women in this study were not only managing multiple and, often, conflicting roles, but were doing this through periods of significant, ongoing, multiple-sourced and recurring grief. Several studies have found increased symptoms of depression as well as incidences of major depressive disorders among parents of children with medical conditions (eg Breslau and Davis, 1986; Blacher et al, 1997; Barnett et al, 2003: 185). Mothers of children with chronic illness are under considerable emotional and psychological distress relating to the care of their child (Redmond and Richardson, 2003: 208). Redmond and

Richardson's study also points to the existence of grief, strain, unhappiness, sleeplessness, inability to concentrate, inability to enjoy daily activities, and depression. I turn now to share stories of grief from the women in this study in an effort to explore new ways of thinking about grief.

Grief from a life changing event

Redmond and Richardson (2003: 209) talk of the 'fragile lives' of those dealing with the combination of complex medical conditions, intellectual disabilities and uncertain life expectancies. I share Tal's (1996: 15) view that trauma and grief can emerge through events that displace one's preconceived notions about the world. Trauma is enacted in a liminal state and is outside the bounds of 'normal' human experience. The individual is left radically ungrounded; reality is torn from their grasp. As Tal reminds us about such a state: there is no substitute for experience – only being is believing (Tal, 1996: 15). The shock of learning of a chronic illness can provoke just such a response (Morse and Johnson, 1991; Vickers, 2001a).

Respondents confirmed their experience of grief from the life-changing event of their child's illness. Sally described the seismic shift in her life when her daughter was born. For most parents, the birth of their child is a joyous time. However, nearly four per cent of parents receive distressing news about their child's health when the child is born. For these parents, the time of their child's birth may become mixed with stress and despair (Quittner et al, 1992; Barnett et al, 2003: 184).

Sally: She was born, and the bottom dropped out of our lives basically. Peter and I were both nurses, both worked in disability. I had the beautiful textbook pregnancy, not a problem. There was nothing to indicate there were any problems ... I can still, to this day, hear my husband's voice saying, because I can remember being on my side recovering from the anaesthetic going, 'Is it a boy or a girl?' – and Peter's got a really deep voice, saying, 'You have to be strong. You have to be strong'. And I'm going, 'Why do I need to be strong? Is it a boy or is it a girl?' 'You have to be strong'. And then he said, 'She's got hydrocephalus' ... hydrocephalus meant a whole lot of different things in terms of here and now, 12 months' time, five years' time, 35 years' time, you know, 100 years' time. (Sally, Interview 1: 9–10; Vickers, 2005c: 208)

Evalyn also shared her radically changed world view, as a result of learning of her son's lessened intellectual development and realising the impact that this was likely to have on his life trajectory, and hers:

> **Evalyn:** [very long pause] The worst thing that happened was that he was actually, when he was 14 months old and he went to see the pediatrician and the pediatrician said that he was developing normally. And he was just, 'He's doing really well'. And then, the seizures started to increase in frequency and you could see a regression. And then you know that … he had suffered brain damage. And so you knew that the path he was taking, which *was* this way [Evalyn indicates with her hand a steep slope upwards] going upwards, has actually flattened out a lot [Evalyn indicates a much flatter slope with her hand]. So, the worst thing is, I guess, giving up the idea of what he was going to be when he grew up and then realising that that's not going to happen. He's actually going to have this sort of a life. And that is really the worst thing. (Evalyn, Interview 1: 52; Vickers, Parris and Bailey, 2004: 42; Vickers, 2005c: 208).

The narratives depict the reality that both Sally and Evalyn's lives were never to be the same. They were both radically ungrounded as a result of a life changing event; their lives had changed forever, in an instant. All parents have fantasies about their children and their child's future (Barnett et al, 2003: 186) and parents experience psychological stress and disappointment when their child does not meet their hopes and expectations. Parents have to let go of and grieve for the expectations and images of their anticipated or 'hoped for' child (Barnett et al, 2003: 186). For Wendy, the changes brought to her and her daughter's life were also traumatic, and life changing, even though the journey to diagnosis of her daughter's rare form of muscular dystrophy was protracted. The shift in their lives was huge; outside the bounds of either of their previous, normal experience. Wendy shared an incident at her workplace where she was unable to respond to a simple question from a colleague about the health of her child. Wendy's familiar and routine life had been so ripped from her grasp that she had not yet learned when, or how, or what, to say to describe it:

> **Wendy:** I saw someone this morning [at work] and they said … 'How's Samantha?' And I think, 'How am I going to answer that?'

And, really, what I want to say is, 'She hasn't been very well lately', but then I don't want to say why. So I haven't found a place around that for myself (Wendy, Interview 1: 28; Vickers, 2005c: 209).

This simple question from Wendy's colleague magnified all that had changed for them both. Larrabee, Weine and Woollcott (2003: 353) discuss the 'wordless nothing' of grief and trauma. For many grieving people, the central question concerning narrating their experiences concerns the very possibility of such a narration. For them, what they have lived is extremely distressing and emotionally disturbing; a complete disruption to normal everyday experience. The assumptions and expectations of what have previously been usual, reliable, humdrum activities are destroyed. They are left with the difficulty of telling the trauma, and of sharing their grief in a way that another might understand, that another can make sense of, and in a way that encapsulates their loss adequately and accurately (Vickers, 2005c). Wendy had not yet found a way to tell her trauma.

Complicated grief resulting from a life-changing event can also result in major depression or generalised anxiety; even post-traumatic stress disorder (Bonanno and Kaltman, 2001: 725–727). Certainly these women repeatedly indicated periods of significant depression associated with their grief, sometimes for extended periods (Evalyn, Polly, Dolly, Sandra, Sally, Wendy, Cate, and Charlene). Polly spoke of the depression that followed her son's chemotherapy to treat his leukaemia, a life threatening form of cancer. For her, the emotional response was *heightened* when the formality of the treatment period ended. She felt bereft and vulnerable, unable to 'do' anything more for her son, yet hoping he would survive. The sense of helplessness and vulnerability Polly shared are frequent accompaniments to the grief experience, especially complicated grief:

Polly: Because, quite frankly, at the end of Thomas' chemotherapy, I think I did have a bit of a breakdown. I was just really depressed and crying all the time. I don't know what happened … You just feel like you're alone. (Polly, Interview 1: 20; Vickers, 2005c: 209)

Charlene also shared her experience of several lengthy periods of depression she had to endure – a black, horrible cloak over her life as a result of her son's paraplegia:

> **Researcher:** Is there anything you feel that you couldn't cope with or you were going to lose the plot or that your life was going to disappear underneath you?
> **Charlene:** I went through depressions.
> **Researcher:** And was it persistent depression? Was it long-term; was it generalised?
> **Charlene:** It was –, I knew I was in a depression. I would put on a good face when I was with the kids, and when I finally got to bed, I could sit in the corner and cry. (Charlene, Interview 1: 13)

What is interesting is Charlene putting on her 'good face', even at home with her children, only allowing the uncontrollable tide of sorrow to flow when in private, in bed late at night, when on her own. Distressed individuals often hide their needs and negative feelings from members of their social network so as not to burden, upset, or scare them off, as well as to ensure that others do not form an impression of them as weak or needy (Silver, Wortman and Crofton, 1990: 400). It is not only at work that people feel constrained in sharing their grief. The next time you are in the presence of another who weeps, notice that, almost without exception, they will apologise for their tears. We routinely see evidence of Western culture bounding – limiting and constraining – open grieving, both at work and at home. Sadly, our culture compels us to apologise for shedding tears.

Ongoing and recurring grief

> **Researcher Note:** *I am writing this file note as a vivid, if painful, exemplar of what these women are dealing with on a routine basis. Today, I arrived at my appointed interview time with Dolly. We had carefully scheduled our second interview and I made my way to the appointed place. When I got there, Dolly's mother answered the door, profusely apologising because Dolly had not been able to get in touch with me, and had been trying to get me all day long. She had not been able to find my number. She had even rung one of the other respondents – Sandra – to get my number. But Sandra was not available and so she couldn't get it from her either. As if she didn't have enough to worry about without also trying to get in touch with me.*
>
> *What had happened, her mother explained, was that Dolly's little girl, Maggie, had had a cold for the last week or so, but didn't seem to be getting any better. I recalled Dolly telling me at our first interview that*

Maggie didn't get colds and was a very healthy little girl (apart from her epilepsy). Dolly must have been very concerned. Given that Maggie had not been getting better, Dolly had taken her to the local doctor early in the afternoon. He had felt it necessary for Maggie to go to hospital. He thought that, rather than a cold, Maggie had low grade pneumonia – rather more serious. So Dolly and Maggie's father had dropped everything to see Maggie into hospital as quickly as possible.

I write this file note deliberately as it so clearly depicts what can happen in these women's working lives. Dolly would have been at work. She would have had to take time off work to pick up her sick child, take her to the doctor, find there was a serious problem, contact Maggie's father, drop everything else (which, I guess, would have included her appointment with me), then try to get in touch with everyone as expeditiously as possible to not inconvenience them. I wonder how many other appointments she'd had to suddenly cancel that afternoon? I wonder how she felt about that? And, importantly, I wonder what was going through her mind with regard to Maggie? She must be really worried.

So here it is: a day in the life of a woman who works full-time and cares for her child with a chronic illness or disability. (Vickers, Researcher Reflections, Monday, 18 August 2003)

This section opens with a reflection that captured the ongoing and recurring nature of the grief these women experienced. The sudden and unexpected illness crisis of Dolly's daughter illustrated how ongoing grief and worry about her child could be triggered, as well as imposing the need to reschedule her workday in an awful hurry.

Chronic grief has been defined elsewhere as prolonged and extended grief, where symptoms are extremely pronounced and the reaction is prolonged and unresolved. The general impression is one of deep and pressing sorrow (Bonanno and Kaltman, 2001: 707). However, this definition focuses on the mourner's behaviour and response. I was concerned, not so much with the mourner's resolution or otherwise of that grief, but with *the ongoing source of the grief*. The grief that these women faced was chronic in the sense that it continued, not because of something the mourner did or didn't do, but because of the nature of *their circumstances*. In this case, the ongoing grief was sourced from their child and events surrounding their child's chronic illness. Raphael (1986: 5) and I (Vickers, 2001a) have both described the personal disaster that accompanies many people's experience with chronic illness. Erikson (1994), when speaking of communities in crisis, also spoke of personal disaster and how it can creep past one's best defences, because of its recurrent, uncontrollable, unanticipated and unbounded nature – the same characteristics I saw here. A personal disaster is:

> One that gathers force slowly and insidiously, creeping around one's defences rather than smashing through them. People are unable to mobilise their normal defences against the threat, sometimes because they have elected, consciously or unconsciously to ignore it, sometimes because they have been misinformed about it, and sometimes because they cannot do anything to avoid it in any case. (Erikson, 1994: 21)

Paradoxical and challenging, ongoing and recurring grief is at once bounded and unbounded, multi-faceted and irregular, in intensity and duration – but always present. Ongoing grief will simmer quietly out of sight, surfacing at a moment's notice when aroused, leaving the bearer bewildered, frustrated and in pain, with their grief 'reactivated', alive and bold, in the foreground of their lives. The grief produces chaos narratives that speak to the uncertainty of every moment (Vickers, 2005a). Everyday, every moment, those living with ongoing grief can be confronted with its recurrence. Wendy described the uncertainty she faced every day with her daughter's illness:

> **Wendy:** Yes, waking early, staying up *very* late, [sigh] tearfulness, lots of loss and grief ... There's no end to it; it's just an ongoing, everyday, 'What's it going to be like?' So it means planning is really hard.
> **Researcher:** Because you don't know what each day is going to bring?
> **Wendy:** No. And she could be fine for five days and then crash. And just when you think, 'Oh good, we've got this sorted – '
> **Researcher:** Something else happens.
> **Wendy:** That's right. You ring up and say, 'Hi! How was your day?' 'Oh, I'm *really tired*, Mum. *I'm bad*'. [imitating a weepy voice] So it's the emotional roller-coaster – the continued uncertainty – I think that's had the biggest impact. And so there's been a lot of grief for me around that. (Wendy, Interview 1: 12–13; Vickers, 2005c: 211)

A notable exemplar of the ongoing and recurring nature of their grief was the concern expressed by these women about the future for their children. Evalyn, Polly, Dolly, Wendy, Sandra, and Sally all spoke with concern about what would happen to their child in adulthood, and who might care for them into old age. This flagged the ongoing nature of their grief; the problems of their child's chronic illness were often not easily fixed, or not fixable at all:

Researcher Note: *As an insider, I find that this 'grief stuff' really resonates with me. There is no doubt that there has been little acknowledgement from those around me of the grief I experience on a regular basis. Certainly, at work, most people (there are a couple of exceptions) just think there is nothing wrong with me. But what is more disappointing is that some members of my own family also assume that nothing much is wrong. Do they want me to detail my anticipation and concern every time I visit the bathroom, go for a walk, try to see into the distance, or decide (consciously) that, yes, for the time being I can continue working full-time? Every time my illness relapses, every visit to hospital, to the local doctor or the neurologist, every time some part of me stops working or gets a little bit worse, I am reminded that my whole future is so uncertain. Actually, the uncertainty exists for everyone, but most people don't recognise it. This fear infiltrates my thinking, planning, mood – my whole zest for living. I try not to let it swamp me but, sometimes, I can't help it, especially during a relapse or following hospital treatment. And I find it so difficult to convey any of this to others. I rarely try. I was unsurprised when it surfaced in these women's stories. I have thought about this often and have written about it previously:*

And how does the knowing witness explain to the 'outsider' the powerlessness and fear – tantamount for this writer – while acknowledging and explicating that the experience of another sick person rests more closely with anger and, yet, for another, in frustration and loss? How might I accurately portray this ubiquitous existence of fear that has been witnessed in others and lived with so closely myself, so that others may truly understand it? How to elucidate this silent and unwelcome 'life-partner' that simmers gently, just below the surface, out of sight to others, yet always within reach for me? How to explain to another who does not have this identity 'additive', this 'schizophrenic' multiplicity of their person? How to explain how it feels to keep at bay something that constantly threatens to overwhelm, to overtake, and to undo? And how can this be tolerable one day and unbearable the next – and how might one accurately convey this? I feel the shackles tighten. I am not even close. The words remain inadequate, the chasm unbridged. (Vickers, 2001a: 137; cited in Vickers, Researcher Reflections, Tuesday, 31 May 2005)

Cate discussed another likely trigger of her grief. She overheard her husband talking on the phone to his mother about his 'disappointment' in their son. I included Cate's experience as ongoing and recurrent grief because I felt that a memory like this, especially if never discussed or resolved, was an issue that was likely to stay with Cate, tainting her feelings and thoughts about her son, her partner, and their respective and collective futures:

> **Cate:** We knew something was up with William. Once I heard him [Colin] say that he was 'disappointed' about it, and that was when he was talking to his mother on the phone, and I heard him say it. And that was kind of hard to hear. (Cate, Interview 1: 20)

Families with children with special needs do experience more marital conflict (Barnett et al, 2003: 185). Cate's experience may have resulted in feelings of hurt and betrayal, leading to a loss of trust in her partner that would have provided an additional source of ongoing grief for her to deal with. Cate's experience depicted one possible outcome of ongoing grief: a life in a constant state of flux and mistrust, with the possibility of things getting much worse quietly surrounding all that she did. Evalyn also expressed this in terms of fear that her son could lapse back to a state of having seizures all the time, seizures which had significantly altered his childhood development, intellectual capacities, and future. She described the fear that stayed with her, even after Kevin had been stable for some time and she had decided to return to work:

> **Evalyn:** When Kevin was so sick and then all of a sudden he was well, because we'd found the right drugs for him, you sort of didn't trust it [laugh]. You thought, 'Oh, he could lapse at any minute'. And, even now, I'm very, very nervous about changing anything about his drug regime. You know, I'm *very, very* cautious. Because I know how bad it can get, and I don't want it to get that bad. (Evalyn, Interview 2: 3)

Wendy, Sandra, Dolly and Evalyn all depicted a trigger for their ongoing grief being a phone call received at work, telling them of a problem with their child. Wendy reported a typical situation in her workday when a call could come, making her heart thump madly. She described her anxiety as a sense of 'oh shit!' (Wendy, Interview 1: 7) anytime her phone rang. When I met with Wendy the second time, I asked her about these phone calls, to learn more about her experience of ongoing grief, especially at work:

> **Researcher:** You mentioned *your* heart racing when the phone rings [at work]. What else do you feel when the phone rings under those circumstances? ...
> **Wendy:** Well, clearly anxiety about Samantha. At that time, we knew less than we know now, and so there was the unknown. So, a lot of anxiety about how long it was going to take to get to her, what was going to happen, etc. The anticipation at certain times when I knew I had commitments that were professional ones, so that concern or anxiety about being interrupted and conflicted in that time. (Wendy, Interview 2: 4)

Wendy was highlighting the ongoing and recurrent nature of her grief. At any given moment – an insensitive comment, a reminder of the future, or an exacerbation of her daughter's illness – Wendy's grief could re-emerge, forcefully and unexpectedly, to be relived. Recurring grief was also characterised by situational reminders that could arise without warning, reminding the bearer of the loss of control in their lives, and of how their lives could change in an instant. Recurring grief resulted in grief re-enacted; lives reassessed; futures reconsidered; pain relived. The difficulty with recurring grief is that it can recur at any time, and is often triggered by changes or requirements of the chronic illness. For example, Oitk's daughter, Belinda (with scleroderma and a wasted right leg), required treatment to lengthen her shorter leg. Belinda was to have a 'cage' attached to her leg, with screws going through her leg, through the bone, with these screws having to be turned several times a day by Oitk to lengthen the leg. This was going to be painful for Belinda; for Oitk, this was not going to be pleasant either – *and* she had to find time around her study and work schedule to inflict pain on her child. Notice Oitk's poignant comment about how she would be dealing with this recurring grief experience alone:

> **Oitk:** She [Belinda] doesn't really realise that it's not going to be much fun, that it's not going to be terribly comfortable. And, I mean, from my perspective, it's going to be hell. Because I'm the one that's got to turn the screws, so I've to inflict pain on her two or

three times a day. [**Researcher:** Oh!] So it's like, 'Good stuff!' [sarcastic]. And I'm not going to have –, I don't have any support (Oitk, Interview 1: 11; Vickers, 2005c: 212).

For Polly, and others, ongoing fears of a recurrence of their child's illness were also reflected. Polly was afraid that her son's leukaemia would relapse, an ongoing fear held alongside concerns about her son's future with Down's syndrome:

> **Researcher:** What are you most afraid of?
> **Polly:** [Pause] Well, relapse, I suppose. [slight pause] You live one day at a time; I don't know. The relapse stuff, you don't want to go there again. But I just feel like *I used* to be afraid of losing the high-powered job; that was my biggest fear – but not any more. (Polly, Interview 1: 38; Vickers, 2005c: 212)

Another of the frequent outcomes of major shifts in one's life is the reassessment of one's priorities. Polly, spoke about just such an adjustment to her own life priorities, realising that her fear of losing a high-powered job was nothing compared to the fear she now held for her son's future health and life expectancy. Vignette 12 was developed based largely on Polly's experience(s) of fear surrounding her child's future survival and healthy development. I developed this to explore how these women might respond to the grief-filled life of another, providing a clue as to how they might want others to respond to them:

Vignette 12: Fear and grief

You are sitting having lunch with a close colleague, a single mum, who has a child with a rare form of cancer. For several years the child has been in remission. You are at the café near your work and having a fun, high-spirited chat, with lots of jokes and fun at your other (less likeable) workmates' expense. You are enjoying your friend's company.

You admire how she copes so well. She seems so strong, so together. She rarely complains about her lot and, if she does, it is always in an upbeat, humorous kind of way. Her child has been through a lot: hospitalisations, drugs, numerous rounds of medical appointments. Your friend has been through it all too and always seems to manage to see the bright side, and find a positive in it all.

You remembered that it is her child's birthday next week. You reach into your bag and pass her a small, brightly wrapped gift for her to give to the child. She bursts into tears.

Through her tears, you gather that her child's cancer has come back. It is very serious. What do you do? What do you think is going on here? What do you say? What do you think her biggest fear is? What do you think might help her the most? (Vignette 12, see Appendix)

I presented this vignette to Evalyn for comment. This is what she had to say:

Evalyn: Hmm. That's upsetting. What do I do? I'd have to give this lady a big hug. That's the first thing I'd do. Because I find that helps, it makes ... a big difference. What do I think is going on here? ... Well, I know how this is; I know how this would be. I mean if Kevin came back and had 10, 15 fits a day, I'd feel exactly the same way. That's like my worst fears are being realised. What do I say? I'd just say, 'You just have to hang in there'. That she's been through it before and she can do it again ... It's just awful. What's the biggest fear? Of course, that the child is going to die – that's the biggest fear. And also the fear of the whole emotional experience again. That's an awful thing that you know you're going to have to go through. You just have to be there for this person. And I think that's what you have to do, is just to be there. Let her talk to you and let her know that you're thinking about her a lot. (Evalyn, Interview 2: 17)

A number of important issues arose in Evalyn's comments. First, even though her child doesn't have life threatening cancer, she could immediately empathise with what the woman in the vignette might have been feeling. There was little hesitation in her response – she *knew*, which confirmed for me the importance of acknowledging the transferability of many of these women's grief experiences, even if their children had different chronic illnesses. Secondly, Evalyn talked about the mother's fear for her child's life but, also, that this mother would have to go through the exhausting and personal emotional journey that attached to such events. Evalyn was concerned about this and oriented herself firmly towards the need to 'be there' for the person in the fictional vignette, especially with regard to the need to help them cope with the inevitable emotional and grief-related challenges that lay ahead. Evalyn had clearly and immediately empathised with this fictional person, placing herself in her shoes.

I also asked Oitk to respond to this vignette. She also was able to immediately empathise, but added another view that I had not anticipated. I believed this was born of her experiences providing support, and receiving support from others. Like Evalyn, her immediate response was to give the person in the vignette a hug. She also empathised with the fictional mother's worry. She knew, without hesitation, that this mother would need support. However, she also recognised her own limitations in being the one to provide that help, especially on an ongoing basis, given her own multiple responsibilities. Finally, she also pointed to her need to be able to stand alone to deal with whatever happened in her life:

> **Oitk:** I'd probably put my arms around her and give her a big hug. What do I think is going on here? She's *worried*. What would I say? Probably not a lot. [slight pause] What do you think her biggest fear is? The child's going to die. And what do you think might help her the most? Has she got other kids? Yes, being around is what's going to help the most and helping out and listening and being at the hospital and doing all that stuff. And you do it for some people and you don't do it for others. There *are* people I would do it for, and there are people I have done it for, and there's people that you just can't. I don't know if you get to that, but I actually get to the point at times that I'd love to help and I just can't.
>
> **Researcher:** Well, there's only so much we can do, isn't there? You have to survive your own set of circumstances. Yes, I'd feel exactly the same sometimes. I wish I could do more but I just have to survive myself.
>
> **Oitk:** I've actually just recently had exactly that. And, also, it's one of those things where you'd help through the hospital bit, but then there is actually a time where you also have to take your hands off it as well and say, 'This is your life. I'm here.' But you can't carry someone through. It's one of those things where sometimes what doesn't break us makes us stronger, so you actually do have to let somebody do it, but you've got to be around. I mean, just *knowing* that there's people there – or having a meal delivered, that kind of stuff – is often more important than the tangible things, rather than being around all the time or being in their face *all the time*. That can actually be as stressful the other way if you're not careful … But in the emergency time, like in that real crux time, yes, you do it for

sure. And, look, I know for me personally, in my life, when people have taken a step back, it has been actually the best thing. Because what happens is, when you get past that initial pressurised time, then if you've got people doing too much for you, you'll let them. And it's actually just harder for you when you have to eventually do it for yourself. (Oitk, Interview 2: 17–18)

Fascinating in Oitk's remarks was evidence of her having previously lived in a situation where people had stepped back from her, when she had needed help. Her response, now, towards helping another similarly placed, was one of ambivalence. She certainly recognised the need for giving support, but seemed to also have learned (the hard way?) the value of people keeping their distance, especially over the long-term. She argued that she had *benefited* from being allowed to do things for herself, and to learn to manage on her own. This vivified Oitk's experience and meaning of surviving, on her own, in an individualistic culture. I believed that she had experienced support being withdrawn from her at some point in the past, and had learned, as a result, to depend on herself and cope alone in order to survive.

Multiple sources of grief

Another of the issues that emerged when speaking to respondents was the number and magnitude of traumatic and grievous events that they had lived and were living, in addition to having to cope with working full-time and caring for their child with chronic illness. We know that women in this situation recognise their own multi-tasked roles (Redmond and Richardson, 2003: 209). However, there has been little acknowledgement of the multiple sources of grief that people often endure in addition to the ongoing and recurrent grief that is directly related to their child. These women had lots of other things to grieve over and worry about that was not being acknowledged.

For example, we know parents of children with ADD are often worried about their children's educational and employment possibilities in the future. Uncertainty and fear about the future is a constant worry for parents of children who are chronically ill (Melnyk et al, 2001). Sandra's son had demonstrated severe anger management episodes that had destabilised her family. We know that nearly half (49 per cent) of children with ADD will experience profound or severe restrictions on their lives, requiring some form of assistance (ABS, 2002: 5). Sandra had much to mourn surrounding her son's challenges with ADD. However, in addition to her son's ADD-related losses and difficulties, Sandra also shared numerous other sources of grief in her life: she had recently lost her father; she was now dealing with a grieving son, who had lost a great source of comfort in his grandfather; she had to care for her mother after her father's death; her mother had broken a bone in her back, preventing her from walking, and also had Parkinson's disease; Sandra had to continue to manage Edward's numerous school changes (including problems with his current school); she continued to manage her business (and the family's primary source of income) during a period of industry downturn; and dealt with significant sibling conflict between her two children (Sandra, Interview 1: 10–11). These events, on their own, were all potential sources of grief. But Sandra had to deal with *all of them at the same time.* Cate also reported multiple sources of grief: guilt feelings about her child's autism; feeling alone with her overwhelming responsibilities; and wondering if her husband blamed her for their child's disability. She spoke, in particular, of the difficulties in her relationship with her partner around the time of her son's diagnosis with autism. Cate made it very clear that, like Dolly and Sandra, she and her husband had not been communicating openly about their respective grief experiences. As a consequence, Cate felt very alone:

> **Cate:** I think that in the beginning it was really hard for me ... there were a lot of worries ... we had a lot of hard times. My husband and I had hard times with each other for a while. And particularly after he was diagnosed. The funny thing about it was that we didn't talk about it – and we still haven't to this day – and the big thing that I worry about is that he thinks it's my fault, because I have a brother [with a disability]. And I've never asked him, 'Do you think it's my fault?' If he ever says it's my fault, that's it. I'll be like, *that's it!* But it never happened. (Cate, Interview 1: 13; Vickers, 2005c: 213)

Dolly also reported many sources of grief. She had recently separated from her partner, who she had learned had been having an affair with another woman for most of the duration of their marriage. Dolly's partner was now living with his long-time girlfriend, just around the corner from Dolly's home. So, Dolly had to deal with: the loss of her partner; her own likely sense of betrayal; Maggie's intellectual difficulties; caring for Maggie on her own; a falling out with her mother; and all the while, she continued to work in a business partnership with her estranged husband. She spoke frankly about the difficulties of balancing her emotions around all these events while still having to care for her intellectually disabled daughter on her own. She shared feelings of guilt, saying that she hadn't dealt with her child's disability 'well', and worried that her daughter would never marry and have children of her own. Dolly grieved the loss of never being a grandmother and of possibly never raising a normal child (Dolly, Interview 1: 9). Dolly shared her unspoken, cherished dreams for the future:

> **Dolly:** I felt bad ... I felt I wasn't dealing with it as well as he [Steven] was. He was ... well *outwardly* he was doing this great thing about, I'd say, 'I'm never going to be a grandmother, and I'm never going to see her get married; she's never going to have children'. And he was being very sensible, saying things like, 'Well, that's just your measures of success. Maggie's measures will be different. It's just having a good life'. Which was all absolutely right ... [but] when we went into personal counseling for our marriage, back in July/August, he completely cracked up. And it all came out that he hadn't actually coped with it at all. And there was this great watershed of emotion that both of us had never really dealt with. And in a lot of ways, yes, I think that has had a bearing on us ...
> **Researcher:** So when it all broke years ago, and Margaret [Maggie] first got sick and in hospital, were you talking about it a lot?
> **Dolly:** Yes, we were talking about it, absolutely. I mean, my husband –, my ex and I have a very strong friendship, still today have a very strong relationship. But I think emotionally we've drifted apart. He apparently had someone else in his life for 15 years, I didn't know about, who'd been a friend and a lover from a previous life, and she'd sort of been doing a bit of a 'Camilla Parker-Bowles' there in the background [indicating they had been having an illicit affair]. And when he was going through all this drama, *he was talking to her*. So he would talk to me, but he would also talk to *her* ... Like, he was talking to her about it. (Dolly, Interview 1: 19–20; emphasis in original).

Parents imagine the kind of person their child will become, the relationships they will have, and the pride and joy they will experience as a parent (Barnett et al, 2003: 186). Dolly was grieving the losses that were a normal part of the attachment process. Her hopes for her daughter, for the future, and of a life with children and grandchildren, had been crushed. Dolly also talked about her multiple sources of grief from the perspective of not having sufficient guidance or support in getting help to manage and deal with her grief. She shared how, while her husband and she were both mentors and coaches to others in their professional lives, no-one thought (including themselves) that *they* should be seeking help to deal with the changes that Maggie's disability brought to their lives:

> **Dolly:** I suppose, more than anything, I hadn't really talked to anybody other than my husband and, even with him, ironically perhaps that's part of the problem with him and I, we didn't talk enough about how we really felt about Margaret's condition. The impact that it really did have on us, we didn't talk about it ... So we probably haven't gone through the kind of grieving, and all the stages you need to go through, when you have something like this. (Dolly, Interview 2: 1–2)

Polly also shared her experience of multiple sources of grief. She reported her experience of reliving her grief at a community healthcare centre, as a result of the thoughtless and insensitive comments of one of the workers there:

> **Polly:** We were talking, and she was saying, 'Were you shattered when he was born?' And I said, 'Well, you get over it'. And she said, 'I would have had an abortion'. You know, if I was a different kind of woman, and if it was a different kind of day, you'd get into a car and drive to the Gap and go off the edge. For all she knew, I was *that close* [indicates closeness with her fingers] to having an abortion and then jumped off the table and ran out. *For all she knew!* (Polly, Interview 1: 42; Vickers, 2005c: 213).

Many of the respondents also shared a sense of a disrupted future, a classic grief response (Bonanno and Kaltman, 2001: 716). Sandra shared her fears for Edward's future, specifically that he might have harmed himself or committed suicide (Sandra, Interview 1). She was upset when discussing it during our first meeting. I gently asked her about it again, when we met the second time:

> **Researcher:** Has something happened to make you be specifically afraid of that [suicide]?
> **Sandra:** I just know when I was a teenager, I had very dark periods where you'd think that life wasn't worth living. And it's a common

thing within teenagers. I don't believe I visibly demonstrated the signs of very little self worth, which Edward has. You just know that kids that don't like themselves, that don't think they're worthwhile, that don't think anything they do –, there's no hope. I don't know why, but I just have this awful intuition. And I'm not a melodramatic or a dark side person. (Sandra, Interview 2: 16–17; Vickers, 2005c: 214)

Wendy also had many sources of grief in her life. She told me about her mother, who had Alzheimer's disease, and her fears that this might be her fate for the future. She also shared that she had a father, who she could not stand, and an estranged husband whom she found, mostly, to be very unsupportive. For many of these women, the multiple sources of grief they experienced added to their concerns for their children. Wendy explained to me that Alzheimer's disease was a genetic condition, predisposing Wendy to the same possible outcome. I wondered how she felt about that. Did she worry about it? Did it influence her experience with her daughter's serious illness? I asked her about this when we met the second time:

Researcher: How much has the situation with Samantha dredged up fears about your health in the future? You talked about your mother having Alzheimer's. For me, health crises in other people trigger fears for myself, and I wondered if you have the same experience?
Wendy: From my mother, yes, because there was the genetic issue. That's been something that's concerned me for a long-time ... I think that was more my concern ... that I could be in a wheelchair and Samantha could be in a wheelchair, and we could both have to look after each other and, 'My God, how are we going to do that?' (Wendy, Interview 2: 8–9)

Wendy also discussed another potential source of grief for her: her other daughter. The possibility of a sibling's discomfort and anxiety surrounding chronic illness has been noted (Murray, 1998). In this case, Samantha's sister Leanne, was very insensitive about Samantha's illness and prognosis. Wendy articulated a complete absence of understanding and empathy from Samantha's sister, regarding the extent, severity and potential consequences for Samantha in the future:

Researcher: And [during the first interview] we go on further talking about Leanne, your older daughter. That Leanne doesn't see Samantha

104 *Working and Caring for a Child with Chronic Illness*

when she's really tired and really sick. There's a sense then that Leanne thinks you're constructing how sick Samantha is …
Wendy: Well, that's true, but that comment also is partially incorrect. Her sister was also at the hospital when she was having the carpopedal spasms. So this sister has actually seen her in great pain and in a really bad condition and, yet, I've received an email from her sister saying that I'm 'catastrophising her illness'; I'm using it to keep her home and keep her bound to me when she ought to be flying. Her sister has such a lack of empathy … But I think illness plays into family dynamics in ways that make it much more painful than the condition itself.
Researcher: Yes, it magnifies all of those dynamics, doesn't it?
Wendy: Absolutely. (Wendy, Interview 2: 7–8)

As an 'insider' to how illness can magnify (sometimes negatively) family dynamics, and as one who has lived the experience of others minimalising and trivialising my experience of illness, I could really relate to Wendy's comments here. There is no doubt, from my experience as a person with MS, that the experience of grief and loss can be heightened immeasurably by a lack of acknowledgement by important others. I know that people look at me and think that nothing very much is wrong. They have so little understanding of: (a) what is actually wrong that they can't observe; (b) how much worse it might easily (and probably will) get in the future; and, (c) how much of a concern this is to me, on a daily basis and, especially, during a period of exacerbation. There has been, from my perspective, little acknowledgement from some family members of just how serious and fear-producing these experiences can be. Wendy also flagged another unanticipated and largely unacknowledged grief outcome, which added to her multiple sources of grief that had resulted indirectly from her daughter's illness. She spoke of the loss of a professional friendship. She talked about the change in a professional relationship with one of her colleagues. This, she explained, was not something she had anticipated and found very difficult to deal with – and at a time when she had so much going on with the journey to her daughter's diagnosis (Vickers, 1998; Vickers, 2001a):

Researcher: But the relationship has changed because of what's happened with Samantha, is that right?
Wendy: I felt that the relationship changed, yes. However, now that the divide's clearly been singled out, the relationship is now almost back. But we don't mention much about our kids. I think it was

their need to place a boundary around, 'I don't wish to be perceived in that role'. Which is understandable; it's about managing different dynamics. But it was quite hard at the time.

Researcher: Yes. Can you tell me about the specifics of your discomfort in that situation? When you say uncomfortable, what does that mean to you?

Wendy: It means uncomfortable because of the assumption that I might have thought of them as a counselor, which they *have been*. Looking at it from their point of view, I guess it would be a way of them protecting themselves ... But it was uncomfortable because I thought it was a step away from a nice, easy, open, uncomplex relationship. In other words, Samantha's disease brought complexity into our ... friendship. (Wendy, Interview 2: 5)

One of the problems that parents of children with chronic illness face is being less able to rely on common sources of social support; friends and family members are often unsure how to help and may avoid becoming involved altogether (Barnett et al, 2003: 185). Wendy's colleague's apparent withdrawal may well have been as a result of their uncertainty as to exactly how they should behave or of wanting to avoid becoming overly involved in her problems. Certainly, the withdrawal of friendship can be particularly painful and is, unfortunately, quite common (Garwick et al, 1998: 669). Cate reported a similar experience (discussed in Chapter 3), where her colleagues stopped talking to her about her child after they learned that her child had autism. Such incidents represent the many and varied – the multiple – sources of grief in these women's lives. Most would not consider professional relationship changes to be a source of grief. However, I claim that it can be and that the resulting grief is unlikely to be sufficiently understood or acknowledged. It is bounded grief.

Grief is always among us, even at work, and it interplays between work and home. I hope to have highlighted the experience of grief lived after a life-changing event, experienced as ongoing and recurrent, or being multiple-sourced. At any time, reminders of grief might arise, at home or at work. Sadly, many fail to recognise the process of grieving and adaptation, especially for parents with a child with chronic illness. Noppe (2000: 523) proposed a 'post-modern' orientation to grief, which allows respect for the diversity of responses to death, and sensitivity to the griever's location in time and culture. I agree, adding that attention to the grieving individual's circumstances is also required.

5

Cruelty and Indifference

Not What I Wanted to Hear

Before she had facial reconstructive surgery
People with jaws to the ground
The whole family, over for a viewing
Look, look, look; point, point, point!
Unbelievable.
Tell them to piss off.

Little old lady asked if I'd hit her
Another little old lady: 'Did you hit her?'
The ice cream man: 'What happened to her?'
A religious man, going on about God
Not something I wanted to hear
I think God sucks at the moment.

(Sally, Interview 1: 22–23)

The data poem created from Sally's story introduces what I believe to
be a significant, and painful, issue that arose in the stories of the
women in this study. In the pages that follow, the theme of cruelty
and indifference is explored. I was shocked at the insensitive, thoughtless and cruel incidents reported. This cruelty came from those closest
to them, partners and family members, as well as those less proximate;
colleagues, friends and even complete strangers. Sally's experience,
introduced in the data poem above and explored in detail below, came
from strangers in her life: people in a shopping mall, someone walking
down the street, a serviceman working in her home. I was floored.

I commence the chapter by examining the construct of cruelty; what
cruelty might be and what possible reasons might exist for people to be

cruel to others. Then, in the stories that follow, I consider examples of cruelty and indifference in ascending order of proximity to the respondent concerned. Incidents were reported from:

- Strangers;
- Colleagues;
- Friends;
- Family members; and,
- Partners.

Strap yourself in.

Narratives of cruelty and indifference

There is little literature available about the construct of cruelty; there is none that talks about cruelty towards parents of children with chronic illness. Indeed, there have only been two empirical studies that particularly address the construct of cruelty (see Kemp, Brodsky and Caputo, 1997; and Caputo, Brodsky and Kemp, 2000: 652). The literature that discusses cruelty tends to be more routinely associated with phenomena other than caring and working, such as: childhood animal cruelty (eg Miller, 2001); abusive family contexts (Duncan and Miller, 2002); child abuse (Reiniger, Robison and McHugh, 1995; Labbe, 2005); adult violence (Duncan and Miller, 2002); inhuman medical treatment (Steele and Chiarotti, 2004); interpersonal aggression, bullying and violence (Klama, 1988; Neuman and Baron, 1997; Laabs, 1998; Felson, 2000; Vickers, 2001c; Hutchinson et al, 2005a; 2005b; 2005c); as well as the numerous very 'efficient' means of invoking harm to others, such as genocide, military massacres, rape, torture and mutilation (Amnesty International, 1975; Mann, 1996; Dutton, Boyanowsky and Bond, 2005).

The construct of cruelty is, then, elusive despite its widespread descriptive use (Caputo, Brodsky and Kemp, 2000: 649). To try and understand the term better and to see if this was the term I sought to encapsulate what these women had reported, I consulted the *Collins Dictionary of the English Language,* which defines 'cruel' as: (1) causing or inflicting pain without pity, or (2) causing pain or suffering (Wilkes, 1979: 359). Similarly, 'cruelty' is defined as the deliberate infliction of pain or suffering, with the quality or characteristic of being cruel (Wilkes, 1979: 359). However, I found other definitions to be more expansive. *The Oxford Encyclopedic English Dictionary* (OED, 1992; cited by Caputo, Brodsky and Kemp, 2000: 650) includes four related definitions for 'cruel': (a) disposed to inflict suffering, indifferent to or taking pleasure in another's pain or distress; (b) fierce, savage; (c) severe, strict, rigorous; and, (d) causing or characterised by great suffering, extremely painful or distressing. What is of interest to me in this latter definition is the addition of the notion of indifference that may be involved in causing distress.

Motivations for cruel behaviour have also been debated. Some believe, dating back to Aristotle, that people are cruel to exact revenge in response to pain they themselves have received (Caputo, Brodsky and Kemp, 2000: 650). The revenge may be directed towards the person responsible for causing the pain or, equally, towards others who have had no responsibility for the original hurt, involving events much later in life. This delayed revenge view conceptualises cruelty as a pathological product of early suffering and accumulated anger; cruel people hurt others as a result of their own past pain (Caputo, Brodsky and Kemp, 2000: 651). This thinking applies equally to aggressive criminals who have suffered childhood abuse (Kellert and Felthous, 1985; cited in Caputo, Brodsky and Kemp, 2000: 651) as it does to neglect or hurt experienced in infancy, through premature separation or other causes, and the subsequent emergence of the cycle of deprivation (Bowlby, 1946; cited by Rustin, 2000) transmitted via deficits in parenting capacity (Rustin, 2000: 165).

A very different explanation of cruelty is that such behaviour is natural or otherwise healthful. This view encourages the belief that all people have dispositions towards inflicting pain on others. Cruel behaviour is regarded as a natural occurrence and (a) only legal or social conventions restrain these natural urges, but that (b) this urge may be unleashed if circumstances permit (Caputo, Brodsky and Kemp, 2000: 651). Some of the circumstances shared in this chapter might well represent these kinds of contextual factors; for example, cruel acts taking place because there was no witness to the cruelty, or no punitive outcome likely. When I reflected on Sally's experiences (introduced in the data poem above), I considered the likelihood of punishment for anyone involved was very remote, potentially having contributed to the perpetrators' hurtful acts.

However, the dominant view (according to Seabright and Schminke, 2002: 28) about immorality – which includes cruelty – stems from a lack of attention, reasoning, or imagination. According to this view, people are cruel or immoral because they just don't give sufficient thought or consideration to what they are doing. Other authors have described this problem in similar ways: Gioia (1992) implicates the failure to think carefully about what one is doing with moral oversight; Rest (1994) attributes unethical behaviour to a deficiency in at least one of the four basic psychological processes – moral sensitivity, moral judgement, moral motivation and moral character; Bird (1996) uses the metaphor of moral silence, deafness and blindness, to explain corporate misdeeds; and Werhane (1998; 1999) argues that moral amnesia stems from a lack of moral imagination (all cited by Seabright and Schminke, 2002: 28). These authors all explain acts of immorality – including cruelty – as being purely a result of the thoughtlessness and lack of attention by the perpetrator towards the person targeted.

One further explanation of cruelty that is of interest to me is that cruelty can involve pleasure for the perpetrator causing the pain. It is not about revenge but about causing pain to another without remorse and without necessarily having a reason. One way to define cruelty under these circumstances might be to consider the awareness and enjoyment that perpetrators may feel about pain intentionally inflicted on others (Caputo, Brodsky and Kemp 2000: 652). Seabright and Schminke (2002: 19) confirm their view that acts of immorality can involve a good deal of thought, attention and consideration. For example, they liken workplace deviance to behaviour intended to harm the organisation or its members, and include in their discussion behaviours such as aggression, retaliation, revenge, and sabotage (Seabright and Schminke, 2002: 20). The bullying literature also confirms this kind of thinking (eg Mann 1996; Vickers, 2001c; Hutchinson et al, 2005a; 2005b; 2005c) and, while bullying was not routinely reported, it was in evidence. Wendy, in particular, commented on being bullied in her workplace and, given her circumstances – that were known to the bullies – I found her shared experiences of bullying and cruelty to be horrible, even unthinkable, given her personal difficulties. Whatever view or understanding of cruelty is preferred, the cruelty and indifference experienced by these women deserved further consideration.

Finally, it is not my intention to presuppose the actual motivation for the cruel and thoughtless acts reported. I do make some assertions of what *might* have been happening, based on my interpretations of the circumstances that these women reported, in order to explain what might have been going on and to draw attention to the painful outcomes that resulted. What concerned me the most was the frequency of such incidents, and the number of areas of their social networks from where they emanated. It also appeared that some were deliberate.

Whether the act was one of indifference to the feelings of the other, of being unconcerned about the likely pain and torment that would have resulted, or whether the acts were intentional and designed to cause harm, I believed them to be cruel.

Finally, I share synonyms of 'cruel' found in *The Macquarie Encyclopedic Thesaurus* that resonated with me when I was thinking about what I had witnessed. Terms included: unkind; cutting; unpitying; ill-willed; spiteful; malicious; mean; nasty; poisonous; venomous; harsh; heartless; inhumane; merciless; pitiless; unsympathetic; brutal; brutish; vicious; and savage (Bernard, 1990: 424.4). Even the phrase 'to act unkindly' gave pause for thought with relevant synonyms being: to do someone a bad turn; bully; abuse; victimise; torment; harry; hurt; maltreat; ride roughshod over; and brutalise (Bernard, 1990: 424.5). It is with these terms in mind that I consider stories of cruelty.

Cruelty and indifference: from strangers

Many incidents characterised as cruelty or indifference came from strangers. Seabright and Schminke (2002) confirm that cruelty often arises in situations where there is no likelihood of punishment for the perpetrators and no likelihood of the cruelty being witnessed. Many of the incidents Sally shared fitted this description. Strangers staring and pointing at her daughter in the shopping mall were largely hidden by their anonymity in the crowded mall. It was also highly unlikely than any punitive response would have been forthcoming. Other incidents, many and varied, also stemmed from situations where either no-one was around to judge the behaviour or, if it was witnessed, it was unlikely to be punished. I was surprised at just how many and how easily Sally could relate these situations. They just tumbled out of her mouth:

> **Researcher:** Has there been any particularly negative situations to do with Nadine's condition which spring to mind?
> **Sally:** [Laughter] Well, I guess I've had things like – probably before she had any cranio-facial reconstructive surgery – we get used to [how she looks], but you could see other people with their jaws to the ground. You'd be at [a large suburban shopping mall], and the kids would drag the whole family over for a viewing, going, 'Look, look, look'! Point, point, point. It was unbelievable.
> **Researcher:** And what did you do when that happened?

Sally: I just thought, 'Oh, whatever'. But I was lucky, because Nadine had well-developed language really, really young. It wasn't just language that I could understand; it was stuff that anybody could understand. So it was good, because she'd come and say, 'They're looking at me'. And I'd say, 'Well, you go over and say, "My name's Nadine. Hello"'. And you'd just see these people freak; they'd scarper or they'd turn bright red on the spot with embarrassment. I can remember there was this little old lady who asked me if I'd hit her. I just was stunned and went, 'No'. Then only two weeks after that, I had another little old lady say to me, 'Oh, did you hit her?' And I just went, 'Yes, the sledge hammer missed her forehead and got her nose'. Like, duh.
Researcher: It's just so appalling – ...
Sally: [Laughter] And the ice-cream man. When I was buying ice-cream: 'Oh! Oh! What happened to her?' It was like, 'She was born like that. You can stick your ice-cream!' Depends on whether I'm having good days or bad days whether I ... just tell them to piss off ... I had this *delightful* [sarcastic] old man come and quote for my awnings. Nadine was asleep and then she woke, and I said, 'I just need to go and get my baby'. He was obviously a religious man, I think, and he sort of said, 'The devil works in mysterious ways. He's certainly thrown a spanner in the basket here'. And I just thought, 'You've got to be kidding me'. And I said, 'It's rather unfortunate for her. I'll get on with life and get on with it, but she has to endure and look like this for the rest of her life'. Because he was going on about God, and I said, 'Well, I think God sucks at the moment, because this little kid has to endure this stuff all the time'. But that kind of, 'Well, God's chosen you because you're obviously a very special person'. She was only a few months old; it certainly wasn't anything I wanted to hear. I just thought, 'Don't give me that shit!' (Sally, Interview 1: 22–23; Vickers, 2005b)

Garwick et al (1998: 669) confirm that strangers are inclined to make insensitive or invasive comments that are hurtful to parents. Staring at the child is also reported as the most common nonverbal source of nonsupport (Garwick et al, 1998: 669). Unlike Garwick and colleagues, I believe that staring and pointing at someone's disabled child is worse than being 'nonsupportive' – it is cruel and completely indifferent to the feelings of both mother and child. What was particularly disturbing about Sally's story were the number and voracity of ugly and cruel incidents that she could bring to mind on the spot. She did not pause;

she did not have to think about the question. She was able to rattle off numerous very hurtful incidents, without any difficulty at all.

Researcher Note: *I admired Sally's ability to laugh about these horrible people. I wondered what I would have done? When I first met Sally, I was using a walking stick because of problems with balance and co-ordination which sometimes made walking difficult for me. I knew, from first hand experience, that people stared at me – a lot – when I used my cane. I recall, outside of the formal interview, laughing with Sally about how people could be so rude and would stare at people with disabilities. I remember we were 'categorising' the different forms of rudeness that accompanied staring. My rough recollections of our shared taxonomy remind me, first of all, of the 'direct stare' type. This is the person who just stares at you (or your child) full on, without trying to disguise their rudeness. Then there was the 'whip around' type. This was the person who walked past you, deliberately not staring; then, when they had gotten far enough past you that they thought it was safe to look, they would quickly turn back to stare at you – long and hard – they thought, without observation. These people obviously had no clue that most of us have peripheral vision. Sally and I also laughed about the 'little old lady' type who we agreed were capable of the worst actions and comments.*

I had certainly found that the little old ladies were the ones most likely to stop me and comment on my walking stick. It was as if they felt that they were 'entitled' to say what they thought about it. I remember when I went to buy my first walking stick. I went to the chemist where they were sold. I was standing there looking at the offerings, not really knowing much about it, how high they should be, which hand one should use, etc. As I was standing there, I asked one such 'little old lady', who had a stick herself, something about what the height of the stick should be. She assumed nothing was wrong with me and looked askance: Rather than answer me she asked, 'Are you getting something done? Are you having an operation?' 'No. I have MS and I have trouble with my balance and with walking sometimes'. She looked completely disbelieving. She also looked at me as if I was mocking her, which I most certainly was not. Mostly, I just found the 'little old ladies' were those most responsible for the 'direct stare' response; the ones I came across clearly felt no discomfort looking me up and down, and curling their lip. It was awful. Obviously, they thought there was nothing much wrong with me and why was I using the stick? Was I trying to attract sympathy? Was I a fake? I have no idea, of course, what they thought. But gauging from the looks on their faces and their body language, they didn't take kindly to someone of my age using a walking stick. If only they knew how much I hated it too! (Vickers, Researcher Reflections, Saturday, 11 June 2005)

Given the obvious need for support in Sally's life, I was astounded by the hurtful comments and behaviours that she had so routinely faced. I would class these as 'societal acts of cruelty' (Caputo, Brodsky and Kemp, 2000: 654). While Sally's experience did not portray acts of persecution directed at issues of religion, race or ethnicity (as Caputo and colleagues suggest), they were acts resulting from another common area of discrimination – disability. Further, the characteristic of the target, in Sally's case, her intellectually disabled daughter, further strengthened the probability of a determination of cruelty. A characteristic of the victim, such as innocence, is a strong contributing factor. People with disabilities and children, in particular, are seen as being innocents, with the corollary being that the degradation of people with disabilities is especially cruel because people with disabilities can do nothing about their situation; it's not their fault (Caputo, Brodsky and Kemp, 2000: 658).

Cruelty and indifference: from colleagues

We have already seen that recognition of organisations being unreasonable and hurtful places is not new. Fromm (1942/1960; 1963/1994), Blauner (1964) and Marx (1975/1994) have all described organisations as alienating places, with the potential to evoke feelings of fragmentation, meaninglessness, isolation and powerlessness (Vickers, 1999; 2005d). There has also been increasing recent recognition of bullying, psychological abuse and aggression in our workplaces (Mann, 1996; Randall, 1997; Neuman and Baron, 1997; Felson, 2000, Vickers, 2001c; Hutchinson et al, 2005a; 2005b; 2005c). The abusive workplace, one that demonstrates little humane concern for its workers, is alive and well (Powell, 1998; Vickers, 2004). I have also, elsewhere (Vickers, 1999; 2001a), highlighted the existence of 'rabid managerialism' as it pertains to the difficulties that exist for marginalised individuals in 'sick workplaces'. Modern workplaces are not conducive to trust and sharing (Vickers, 2005e). However, they *are* conducive to cruelty and indifference.

So, I was surprised when, initially, Evalyn stated that her current workplace was very supportive; she cited specific individuals as being very helpful and supportive, and pointed to the fact that she could work at home when she needed to. She was also comfortable disclosing to her colleagues about her son's disability (as we will see in Chapter 7). However, her ambivalence emerged. Evalyn had also experienced cruelty and indifference at her work. She told me about a colleague who had been completely insensitive to her feelings:

> **Evalyn:** You know, one person –, I didn't really know, one person said to me, 'How could two really intelligent people have a child like Kevin, like yours?' And I was, I just couldn't believe she said that. I was so –, I didn't say anything, I just said, 'Mm-mmm'. And, you know, I just couldn't believe someone said that to me. (Evalyn, Interview 1: 53; Vickers, 2005b)

I returned to this incident during my second meeting with Evalyn, asking her about the context of that comment, so that I might have understood it better:

> **Researcher:** This was when one person said something really horrible to you. [reading the transcript of Interview 1]: 'How could two really intelligent people have a child like Kevin, like yours?' What were the circumstances surrounding that comment? Do you remember?
>
> **Evalyn:** I was working in Finance at the time and I was just starting to get to know some of my colleagues in the group, because I hadn't worked there very long. I had just wandered into one of my colleague's office, and we were just talking about our family situation and life, and I'd mentioned that I had a child with a serious intellectual disability; and that's really how it came up. It was *very hurtful* at the time and I was kind of in shock but I think that's just how that person thinks ...
>
> **Researcher:** If you had your time over, would you say anything different to her? ...
>
> **Evalyn:** No, not really. That was an off the cuff remark ... I don't think she thought she was being nasty. She probably was just insensitive and thoughtless. (Evalyn, Interview 2: 8–9)

Evalyn appeared to be reasonably sanguine about this incident when reflecting on it later, but it had hurt at the time. Evalyn had reported a very flexible workplace policy scenario. However, the literature confirms parents of sick children claim that bosses and coworkers make insensitive remarks (Garwick et al, 1998: 669). In work settings, families have also encountered inflexible work policies that do not accommodate their needs. One report showed a boss saying to a distressed father that he didn't care what was wrong: 'Don't bring it to work' (Garwick et al, 1998: 670). In the stories here, I saw numerous examples of what Garwick and colleagues characterise as unsupportive and unhelpful. However, once again, I interpreted such acts not merely as unsupportive, but cruel and insensitive.

Another hurtful workplace experience was reported by Cate, who reported how her relationship with her colleagues changed, quite dramatically, after her son was diagnosed with autism. I introduced Cate's experience in Chapter 3, when Cate shared how her colleagues had stopped talking to her. I point here to the cruelty associated with that behaviour from her colleagues and include evidence of Cate's colleagues having talked behind her back, while not offering support:

Cate: He was just about to turn two. About three months shy of two. And I knew it inside myself, and some of my coworkers said it too, but not to me. Later on, they said, 'Cate's kid's autistic'. And the funny thing about it was, the one lady who said it first was a lady who worked for me who also had a disability herself. I've got a couple of ladies here who have special needs – they're high functioning – but she *knew it*. And I said, 'How come you didn't tell me or talk to me?' And she just said, 'I didn't know how to say it' ... And one lady who had a kid his age would say, 'Nothing's wrong with him. How could you possibly have a kid with a disability and work here? You're just being paranoid'. Mostly it was 'able me' saying, 'I think something's wrong'. And most people would say, 'There's nothing wrong with him'. You know, they would deny it.[1] And then finally when I went through the whole thing of the evaluations and stuff like that, then I was like, 'William has autism'. Then after that, we didn't talk any more. Now we still don't really talk. People don't really –, we talk a little bit. You know, 'My daughter's going to kindergarten now. She's doing this now'. They'll bring in their kids, and the kids are like, 'Hi, how are you? What's going on?' ... but William says nothing. Nothing. Sometimes I'll bring him in and he'll visit, and they'll visit with him, but we don't talk in an excited way like we used to. And it's OK. It's totally OK.
Researcher: Does it bother you?
Cate: Yes, kind of. It's kind of like you would think that my coworkers wouldn't feel as –, they know me ... And they know about my brother [referring to her adult brother with a disability]. They know they can approach me. (Cate, Interview 1: 21–22; Vickers, 2005b)

We see another example of what Garwick and colleagues (1998) would term unsupportive workplace behaviour, where Cate's colleagues avoided talking about her child's disability (Garwick et al, 1998: 669; Ingram et al, 2001: 175). However, once again, I think this was more hurtful than unsupportive. For Cate, her colleagues conspired to reduce her ability to connect with them emotionally about her experiences of parenting a child with autism, by not speaking with her about it. Cate also described how her colleagues had talked behind her back before Billy's diagnosis, and then stopped talking to her after finding out about his autism. What was extraordinary about Cate's situation was that Cate worked in a centre that supported people with disabilities. One might expect people that work with people with disabilities to be less discomforted with disability generally, and be more responsive and sensitively disposed towards those in need.

However, one can also see the possibility of 'immoral imagination' here (Seabright and Schminke, 2002: 23), where people don't think about what they are doing or the harm that can result. A further possible explanation is that Cate's colleagues are operating 'naturally'; that they felt uncomfortable and didn't know what to do or say. However, Cate was clearly very hurt by her colleagues' behaviour. The literature confirms the distress that parents frequently experience as they realise that their infant looks and responds differently than other babies or is delayed in development (Robson, 1997; Melnyk et al, 2001). Whatever provoked their actions, the result for Cate was very painful.

Sally relayed an incident involving one of her colleagues wanting to gossip about her disabled child, immediately after the child was born. In the passage that follows, Sally described the very traumatic period immediately following the birth of her child. You will recall that Sally's daughter was born with hydrocephalus, lipoma, a significant facial disfigurement and cleft palate, and a significant intellectual disability. We saw in Chapter 4, the grief, stress and despair that can affect parents who receive distressing news about their child's health, especially if their child is born with a serious chronic illness, health defect, disability, sensory impairment, or intellectual disability (Barnett et al, 2003: 184). As one can imagine, Sally had a lot to digest immediately following the birth of her daughter and her colleague's insensitivity and cruelty, especially given Sally's circumstances, was particularly poignant:

Researcher: You've mentioned some special friends that you can obviously really count on. Are there are any friends or colleagues that have particularly disappointed you?

Sally: Yes. One *beautiful* example. [Laughter] This one woman. When Nadine was first born she was transferred to Randwick [hospital]. Because I'd had a Caesarean, I wasn't able to go. I got a day pass on the Wednesday, so I hadn't seen her from the Saturday [when Nadine was born] to the Wednesday, apart from this hideous Polaroid shot I had at my bedside. I can remember Janice, my good friend, saying, 'Chris [one of Sally's colleagues] wants to go and see Nadine'. And I said, 'What for?' And [then] I said, 'She wants to go and have a look!' And I said, 'No!' And it was really interesting that I could even reason at that stage of all the emotional –, I could actually read what she was up to. She wanted to 'stickybeak' so she could go back to work, big note herself, because *she'd* seen the baby – because everybody at work knew ... [Sally replied,] 'I haven't even seen her yet. So no, she can't'. So I went to see [Nadine] on the Wednesday, but the sneaky bitch went on the Friday. She did; she went and did it!
Researcher: Even though you'd said 'No?'
Sally: Yes, even though I'd said 'No'. (Sally, Interview 1: 35; Vickers, 2005b)

We know that the business ethics literature generally attributes unethical behaviour, such as what we have seen here, to a failure of moral perception or reasoning. It is often believed that people don't think before they act and don't consider the implications of their behaviour. However, Seabright and Schminke's (2002: 28) alternative view is to suggest the possibility that misbehaviour, like Sally's colleague's, can be considered an active, even creative process. They propose that a relatively overlooked source of misconduct is an immoral imagination. They argue that an immoral imagination can shape every facet of decision-making: sensitivity; judgement; intention; and implementation (Seabright and Schminke, 2002: 28). Certainly, Sally's experience depicted the immoral imagination of Sally's colleague, implying sensitivity, judgement, intention and implementation that had gone awry – a result of deliberate actions and choices.

The worst work-related experience Wendy reported was a situation where she felt as though she was being deliberately portrayed as someone who was not entirely in control of her circumstances. We know that workplaces can be abusive, inhumane, alienating, aggressive and hurtful places. The bullying literature is replete with a myriad of possible ways and means where negative experiences can be magnified.

One possible way of harming the career of another that bullies often adopt is to portray that person as being 'out of control'. This tactic, especially when directed towards women at work who are vulnerable as a result of a negative life experience, can be very harmful and hurtful to the target, creating even more stress for them to manage. Wendy shared:

> **Researcher:** Have there been any other negative situations [talking about professional relationships]?
> **Wendy:** Yes. I was working at home, but I was working at home *not* because of my daughter ... This [colleague], I believe, has taken substantial liberties with the fact that I had a sick daughter, and used that as a way of explaining why he excluded me in the process of putting in a [competitive professional bid for work], *in my name*, and including my CV, and putting me down as in charge without ever showing me the application. And I'll give you a copy of that email because it positions me as someone who didn't have her mind on the job because I had a lot of things on my plate. And I think he's used and abused that ... I think that's probably the most negative effect (Wendy, Interview 1: 10).

Wendy had previously impressed upon me how long she had been having difficulties with bullying in her workplace. Bullying involves the persistent embarrassment and humiliation of a person (Lewis, 1995: 31). Bullying is deliberate, hurtful and repeated mistreatment of a target, driven by the bully's desire to control the other person (Yamada, 2000: 478). It has even been characterised by some as emotional abuse, as well as hostile verbal and nonverbal, nonphysical behaviours, such that the target's sense of self as a competent person and worker is negatively affected (Yamada, 2000: 478). Those who seek to belittle others in organisations often do so for the fun of it (Gabriel, 1998: 1329). For Wendy to have experienced this during a period of extreme grief and stress, would have been very distressing for her. What is often misunderstood about bullying is that it includes unpredictable, irrational and unfair acts of aggression, violence or abuse (physical, verbal, psychological or emotional) that may include lots of 'smaller events' including the persistent embarrassment and humiliation of a person (Lewis, 1995: 31), exclusion, stereotyping, obliteration of significant identity details (for example, spelling a name incorrectly), rudeness, broken promises, ignoring or keeping people waiting, ingratitude (Gabriel, 1998), professional obstruction, coercion, or setting a person up for failure (Barron, 2002: 153). Bullying includes actions that are vindictive and malicious, and attempt to undermine the target in just the manner Wendy described. Wendy also reported that, while she had been bullied for some time at her workplace, the effects were worse for her when her daughter became ill – exactly what the bully would have intended:

> **Researcher:** Yes. The lack of support you're receiving now is connected with past problems.
>
> **Wendy:** Oh, it's just an ongoing situation with [Wendy's manager].
>
> **Researcher:** Is it worse for you now, given Samantha's illness?
>
> **Wendy:** You mean, is he treating me any worse now because of her illness? Or is my experience of it –?
>
> **Researcher:** Either.
>
> **Wendy:** I don't think he's treating me any worse; he's always treated me badly. But I think my experience of it is that it is more complex now. There's even more at stake. I'd like to be able to stay at [my workplace] for the next 12 months ... there will be an impact, and I'm sure that's a convenient impact to marginalise the direction that I was growing, personally and collectively ... This will be the third occasion that he's attempted to shut down my reinvention of my professional work there. So that has an impact on the consequences of the decisions I need to make in the light of Samantha's illness. (Wendy, Interview 2: 12)

Wendy is clearly articulating her recognition of the cruel and undermining behaviour she has been subjected to over a long period. Despite popular misconceptions, targets of bullies are often outspoken about wrongdoing and are likely to stand up for their own or another's rights. People targeted by bullies are frequently *more attractive, confident, successful, qualified or popular than are the perpetrators*. However, they are often vulnerable for a particular reason, possibly due to illness or as a result of being the sole breadwinner (Gaymer, 1999; Mayhew and Chappell, 2001; Wallis Consulting, 2001). The fact that the bully did not let up on Wendy during the period of her emotional turmoil and grief was cruel, deliberate and intended to harm.

Cruelty and indifference: from friends

Unfortunately, cruelty and indifference doesn't always come from strangers or colleagues. Cruelty may also come from those much closer to us – our friends. Unfortunately, the *majority* of unsupportive behaviours from community members comes from acquaintances, including neighbours, church members, other parents – and friends (Garwick et al, 1998: 669). Insensitive comments, lack of understanding, and inadequate support have all been noted (Garwick et al, 1998: 669). Dolly reported a very callous and insensitive remark about her daughter, Maggie, from her friend:

> **Dolly:** Yes, it was just the most horrific thing. A girlfriend of mine, and I say that extraordinarily loosely [laughter] ... she would always be extremely over the top about Margaret. Oh, you know, 'I don't know how you do it. I don't know how you cope'. ... She rang me one day and said to me, 'Oh, how's Maggie?' 'Oh yeah, she's going quite well'. And, you know, something good had happened at the time and I was feeling quite happy about it, some little improvement. And she said to me, 'You know, sometimes I think it would be better if Maggie just went to bed one night and didn't wake up'. I just couldn't believe it. I mean, I could barely speak. And I said to her, 'I can't talk to you. I have to go'. And I came home – and I'm not a crier – but I just *howled*. (Dolly, Interview 1: 28; Vickers, 2005b)

One can only imagine the pain that this comment caused. A dehumanising approach was evident; Dolly's friend seemed oblivious that they were talking about Dolly's *child*. Dehumanisation divests persons of their human qualities so they are no longer viewed as persons with feelings, hopes and concerns, but as subhuman objects (Bandura, 1990: 28; Seabright and Schminke, 2002: 23). Immoral imagination engenders moral exclusion to dehumanise the other. There was no consideration of the love that Dolly felt for Maggie. Immoral imagination, such as described here, actively excluded Dolly's child, creating a psychological distance, irrespective of the closeness of the original relationship (Seabright and Schminke, 2002: 23). At best, the comment from Dolly's 'friend' arose out of thoughtless indifference. At worst, it was calculated to hurt. Either way, it was cruel and indifferent to Dolly's feelings. Of interest, because of the referral process used to recruit respondents in this study, I also had the opportunity to learn more of Dolly's experience from another respondent. Oitk knew of Dolly's experience also and raised it with me, without prompting, during our second meeting. At the time, I had been asking Oitk to respond to Vignette 2:

Vignette 2: Cruelty, thoughtlessness, managerialism
You are at work, in a meeting with one of your senior managers. You receive a phone call, telling you that your child has been sent home from school/childcare, with a very high temperature. You have previously told this manager of the health problems your child experiences, as you have had to leave work in a hurry previously. You tell your manager what has happened, anticipating a supportive comment and an invitation to leave immediately to see your child. Instead, he proceeds to give you a lengthy lecture about the importance of leaving your 'home' problems at home. He then asks you how often is 'this sort of thing' likely to keep happening?

What do you say? How would that influence your feelings about working there in the future? For example, would you (could you) leave? Would you complain about his behaviour to anyone at work? (Vignette 2, see Appendix)

Oitk had emphasised to me that she had not personally experienced the kind of cruelty indicated in the vignette. However, the vignette raised in her mind Dolly's experience, which was clearly an incident that had resonated with Oitk, almost as much as it had with Dolly:

> **Oitk:** I have never had that by the way [referring to Vignette 2]. I've never ever seen it. Having said that, I've never seen anybody react that way. Not even some of the *horrible* people I've worked with; it's been about horrible other things, not that kind of stuff.
> **Researcher:** Well, I'm very sad to say that most of these are based on true –,
> **Oitk:** On true experiences. That's bad ... This one, actually this one [referring again to Vignette 2], Dolly has had *that* story in *her* life but it was nothing to do with work. A friend told her that she might be better off if her child just died. And in actual fact, the reaction to that was, the four women who were sitting at the table when she told us, were all in tears and we all just welled up when she told us. It was like [sharp intake of breath]. (Oitk, Interview 2: 8–9)

Dolly, who had recently separated from her partner, had spoken of wanting to be in a relationship again. However, thoughtless remarks were also shared with Dolly about her future dating prospects and how they related to her daughter's disability:

Dolly: Interestingly, a number of people have said to me ... 'Are you going to think about dating?' 'Yes'. I really loved being in a relationship. I loved the partnership. I loved being married. And I would like – whether I'm married or not is irrelevant – but I'd really like to go back into a partnership again. And I'd actually like, I'd really love, to have another child. I mean, I'm really running out of time here. But I really actually would like to have another child. I mean, if it happens, it happens; if it doesn't, it doesn't. And someone said to me, well, a couple of people have said to me, 'Oh, it's going to be really hard for you to find someone who'll take Margaret on'. [pause, Dolly shifts uncomfortably in her chair] And one person said, 'If they really love you, you'll know if they really love you if they take Margaret on'.

Researcher: Did you say anything to that?

Dolly: No, I was a bit 'gob smacked' [shocked] to be perfectly honest. (Dolly, Interview 1: 65–66; Vickers, 2005b)

This particular response prompted me to develop Vignette 4, entitled 'Relationships' for comment from respondents. I wanted to know if they thought this was as cruel as I did. I asked Wendy to read the three parts of the vignette, to gauge her response:

Vignette 4: Relationships
PART I

You are a single mum. You have been working at your current workplace for some time. You enjoy your work and are coping as best you can with caring for your child on your own. You have only told one person – in confidence – about your child's illness at your work.

Recently, you have developed a particular friendship with one of your single male colleagues. You like him a lot. The two of you have started to regularly 'do lunch'. You have found, during your discussions, he was married for about three years, but has recently divorced. He has no children from that marriage. He suggests a meal out together and you accept immediately, then retreat into a personal panic, as you wonder who will babysit your child. You also wonder when, and how, you are going to tell him about your child. What do you do?

Wendy (Interview 2) asked, after Part I, 'Why do I need to tell him?' She then read on:

PART II

You ask your very understanding mother to babysit for you – again – on this special occasion. However, she warns that she is 73 and can't be expected to care for your child all week after school while you are working, *and* on the weekends while you go off partying. You go to dinner and have a great time. You decide that you need to tell him about your child but are nervous about his reaction. What do you do?

After Part II, Wendy indicated her belief that her daughter was a major part of her life and she needed to gauge the reaction of this new man in her life to her daughter's condition:

Wendy: The way that I would be orientating myself is: 'I'm a package deal'. If he's the kind of person that has a problem, then he's not the right kind of person for me. (Wendy, Interview 2: 15)

Wendy read on:

PART III

Well, it seems that you don't need to tell him, because your 'friend' at work – who you confided in about your sick child – has already done so. She has been noticing you and 'Mr Right' lunching together regularly, fancied 'Mr Right' herself, and decided to let him in on your 'secret' before you had a chance to. You know this, because Mr Right mentioned it to another person at the office, who then came and asked you if it was 'true what they had heard about your *poor little darling*?' and '*How awful*!' Not only has Mr Right not called or asked you to lunch since you had dinner (this is now two weeks later), you are feeling like an outcast. Everyone is whispering about you, feeling sorry for you, and now talking about your child as if he is some kind of a 'freak'.

As you are leaving the office one evening, Mr Right is leaving at the same time. You ask if he enjoyed your evening out. He is very uncomfortable and says that he has to go. You see Mr Right and your 'friend' lunching together the next day.

How do you feel? What would you do (if anything)? (Vignette 4, see Appendix)

Wendy commented, after reading Part III:

> **Wendy:** Actually, I've had one of the receptionists at work come and do this with me, trying to find out what was going on ... I'd feel very hurt, but I would need to process the fact that he was not Mr Right.
> **Researcher:** Would you do anything or say anything?
> **Wendy:** I'd certainly want to, and I would rehearse all sorts of comments in my head.
> **Researcher:** What about 'your friend' who told Mr Right about your child?
> **Wendy:** That's a good question. It would depend what the nature of my relationship with my friend was, and it would depend on what was at stake. (Wendy, Interview 2: 15)

What I learned from Dolly, Oitk and Wendy was that they believed it was very hurtful for people to be betrayed by friends, however, not so terribly uncommon. Cruelty and indifference, even from friends, is something to be concerned about.

Cruelty and indifference: from family

Social networks can be responsible for up to six types of negative illness-related behaviours: ineffective help; being overly cheerful or optimistic; being overly solicitous; being unwilling to discuss emotional ramifications of the disease; physical avoidance and uneasiness; and resentment (Ingram et al, 1999: 314). Ingram and colleagues (2001: 175) also identify unsupportive acts as those minimising the impact of the event, judgmental behaviour, being overprotective, being overly pessimistic, being rude and insensitive, or having inappropriate expectations about the person's adjustment process. Some researchers have characterised these behaviours as social conflict, conflictual and disappointing experiences in interpersonal relationships.

I found cruelty from family members particularly disturbing. Once again, I found the determination that 'unsupportive responses' were merely 'conflicted' or 'negative' to be unhelpful and euphemistic, when considering the outcome of real human suffering. The closer people perpetrating these negative and unsupportive interactions were to the respondents, and the more central they were to the respondent's lives, the more likely it was that their unsupportive acts were determined to be cruel and indifferent – especially when it was so clear that these women needed help. If families weren't aware and supportive, then who would be?

Dolly reported an argument with her mother that transpired shortly after Dolly and her husband had separated. Dolly explained to me that, after the separation from her partner, she had tried to redefine the various roles in her life – which included taking back some of the care of her child that she believed her mother had been dominating in her carer support role. However, her mother, rather than trying to understand the upheaval, pain and turmoil in Dolly's life at the time, responded in a manner that I considered to be unthinking and cruel:

> **Dolly:** When Steven and I first split up in January, I said to her, 'This is an opportunity for me to have a really clean slate. I'm giving you notice that, at some point, I don't want you to live with me any more'. And she was like, 'You'll never cope. You're a really bad mother. The only reason I stay around here is because Margaret needs me'.
> **Researcher:** How did you feel when she said that?
> **Dolly:** Well, I wanted to smash her [laughter]. The other thing is, when she sold her house at Quakers Hill and came [to live with Dolly] here, she said, 'Here's a gift: one hundred and fifty thousand dollars', which was terrific. It was, 'You're going to get it all anyway when I die', blah-blah. It was helpful, but we didn't need it. Then she did the whole, 'Well, I want the money back then'. I said, 'I thought it was a gift'. 'No!!' ... Anyway, I actually pay her a thousand dollars a month to live away from home now. That's a thousand dollars well spent! (Dolly, Interview 2: 10–11)

It is important to recognise and identify specifically unhelpful, annoying, and upsetting behaviours of others in the social network, including family, and how these behaviours might precipitate arguments and disagreements, and perpetuate negative feelings (Ingram et al, 1999: 314). Sally recounted the absence of any real understanding from her own family and, in particular, her partner's parents. What she described below took place shortly after her daughter, Nadine, was born:

> **Sally:** My parents couldn't really cope. Peter's [Sally's partner] parents I don't think understood at all.
> **Researcher:** Why do you say that?

Sally: They're very religious, so it was all about, 'God will make it better'. And it was kind of like, 'Oh, you just don't get it!' And I guess that's probably really unkind, because I tend to be very practical. While it was devastating and all that kind of stuff, it was, 'Well, here it is; just deal with it and get on with it'.

Researcher: It must have been very – 'distressing' is perhaps a bit too strong – but it must have been very uncomfortable to hear things like that? ...

Sally: I think for them I was, 'Oh, you're just stupid' [laughter]. I just dismissed it. I'm sure Peter's father thought that it happened because I smoked, because I had the odd cigarette.

Researcher: Oh no! It was, 'all your fault?'

Sally: Yes, it was, 'all my fault'. But that's OK. Again I thought, 'If that's what you're comfortable with', you know, 'that's OK'. My parents, I think that for a long time, and probably still now, my father struggled with the imperfection. Because for many years, every phone call was, 'Have you spoken to the plastic surgeon? Have you spoken to the plastic surgeon? She'll be psychologically scarred!' I felt like saying, 'She'll only be scarred because you're going to make her scarred. Nobody else is'. (Sally, Interview 1: 13–14; Vickers, 2005b)

The phenomenon of blaming the parents for the child's condition has also been reported elsewhere (Garwick et al, 1998: 669) and identified as an important source of unsupportive behaviour. Again, I find the term 'unsupportive' a euphemism, minimising the significance of the comments and inferences that Sally had to endure, and the likely hurt it may have caused. Caputo, Brodsky and Kemp (2000: 654) would have termed this 'miscellaneous cruelty', citing examples that don't fit into their other developed categories of cruelty, which include: physical cruelty, sexual cruelty, societal cruelty and ordinary cruelty. Miscellaneous cruelty comprised around 11 per cent of cruel acts reported in their empirical study, and included things like confinement, kidnapping, mental abuse and attempted suicide as an act of revenge. Whether I have correctly categorised Sally's experience, there needs to be recognition that cruelty results in psychological and emotional harm and pain. Implying that Sally was somehow responsible for her child's numerous physical and intellectual disabilities would have, whether intended or not, been responsible for adding to guilt that Sally might already have been feeling after the birth of her daughter. It was also hurtful and cruel.

Cruelty and indifference: from partners

Finally, I explore examples of cruelty from partners. I have reported several incidents in other chapters: Dolly's ex-partner moving in with his long-time girlfriend, just around the corner from where Dolly and her daughter lived; Sandra's partner refusing to take on any emotional load or communicating with Sandra about the problems their son was experiencing – including serious depression – as a result of ADD; Wendy's ex-partner not engaging with their daughter about her condition, even though he was responsible for passing it to her genetically; and, Cate overhearing her partner tell his parents on the phone how 'disappointed' he was with their autistic son (an incident further explored in Chapter 6). Charlene's experience of cruel and indifferent behaviour from her ex-partner [the father of their disabled son] – which was behaviour that had to have been carefully thought out – was to work *against* her, as she struggled to cope with supporting and caring for her two young children. Charlene's ex-partner had run over Jamie as an infant, causing his paraplegia:

> **Charlene:** My ex-husband ran over Jamie. So he was very guilty. He was very nonsupportive of me. When I filed for divorce, he got a lawyer and filed that I was an unfit mother. And the fact that I had shown that the previous five years of income tax, the only person in our household that earned a living was me – that he hadn't worked – helped me. Jamie had a home teacher who had come into our home and wrote a letter saying that she had observed the children at home and that I was a good mother. But I still had to go through court and take care of that. (Charlene, Interview 1: 10; Vickers, 2005b)

In Charlene's case, not only did she have to work three part-time jobs to support her two children, she had to fend off a lawsuit from her ex-partner who was accusing her of being an unfit mother – after *he* had run over their child. One wonders if the revenge that seems to be apparent here – the cruelty – might have emanated from his pain, guilt and anguish resulting from the tragic accident involving his son. Whatever motivated his cruelty, the lawsuit required conscious choices and immoral imagination on his part – cruelty and indifference to his ex-wife's needs – and a recipe for strain and distress for Charlene.

One final point: Caputo, Brodsky and Kemp (2000: 655) noted gender differences in determining what people find to be most cruel. For example, the male participants in their study were more likely than the female participants to cite murder or physical assault as being the cruellest acts. However, the female participants were more likely to cite societal cruelty (acts of discrimination or persecution), or incidents characterised as miscellaneous cruelty, as being the most cruel. A male may read this chapter thinking that the incidents reported were reasonably defined as 'unsupportive' or 'unhelpful'. Conversely, women may be more inclined to consider them as cruel and hurtful, whether deliberate, thoughtless, or in response to their own pain. Whatever the orientation, these stories revealed that these women were subjected to numerous painful life experiences as a result of the cruel (or unsupportive) acts of others. This deserves further thought.

6

Clayton's Support

He Thinks It's My Fault

In the beginning it was really hard
A lot of worries, hard times, after William was diagnosed
We didn't talk about it – we still haven't
My husband, he thinks it's my fault.

(Cate, Interview 1: 14–15)

Introducing 'Clayton's support'

I introduce here what I have termed 'Clayton's support', that is, the support you get when you are not getting support (Vickers, 2005b). This concept borrows from the advertising campaign for a non-alcoholic beverage called Clayton's, where consumers were encouraged to indulge in the drink they could have when not having an alcoholic drink. Clayton's support can be observed as lack of support, withdrawn support, support anticipated but not received, as well as unsupportive and unhelpful behaviour from those in the social network.[1] Parents of children with chronic conditions exist simultaneously within several social networks (eg family, school, community and healthcare) (Garwick et al, 1998: 666). Given that the most beneficial forms of social support are those that match the needs elicited by the particular stressor (Ingram et al, 2001: 174), witnessing Clayton's support was most troubling. Unfortunately, all respondents confirmed the existence of Clayton's support; from partners, family, friends, colleagues, or professionals working with their child. The gap between anticipated or desired support was evident in both work- and home-related circumstances. Where a gulf existed between what support might have been expected – or what had been promised – and what actually transpired, problems emerged. An example of unsupportive behaviour reported by Cate – and illuminated in the data poem above – was that of her husband avoiding communicating with her about their son, William, and his autism. Avoiding communication about important concerns has been classified elsewhere as unsupportive behaviour (Ingram et al, 2001). I call it Clayton's support.

Numerous studies have documented the unique emotional and physical demands that stress and strain parents raising a child with chronic illness (for example, Bruce et al, 1994; Florian and Findler, 2001; Barnett et al, 2003). In addition to the normal stressors associated with having a child, parents of a child with chronic illness also have to cope with many uncertainties surrounding their child's health and prognosis, including attendance to frequent medical appointments and procedures, and the additional workload of caring for a child with special needs (Barnett et al, 2003: 185). Unfortunately, in many instances reported here, needs were not met. Indeed, the reverse was often true. In many instances, negative life events were not only unsupported, but responses were unhelpful and far removed from what might have normally been anticipated.

There is ample research on the effects of social support and its potential to help an individual adjust to stressful situations more successfully (Argyle, 1989: 277; Blaney and Ganellen, 1990: 300; Dunkel-Schetter and Bennett, 1990: 267; Hobfoll and Stephens, 1990: 454; Sarason, Sarason and Pierce, 1990: 10; Silver, Wortman and Crofton, 1990: 397; Hastings, 1992: 236; Ray, 1992; Roskies, Louis-Guerin and Fournier, 1993: 618–619; Garwick et al, 1998; Ingram et al, 1999; Ingram et al, 2001; Barnett et al, 2003). Social support from social networks buffers the negative effects of stressful events and enhances physical and emotional well-being in adults (Garwick et al, 1998: 665). Psychosocial resources such as perceived control, the ability to utilise social support, and the ability to cope with stress are important to help parents survive (Barnett et al, 2003: 186) and can be bolstered significantly by the social network.

Parental coping and perceptions of control have also been found to buffer or protect parenting sensitivity and well-being from the deleterious influences of stress (Barnett et al, 2003: 186). Social support is very important and its lack was definitely an issue for the women in this study. While Garwick and colleagues (1998) identify several social systems existing in the lives of parents with children with chronic illness, such as family, school, community and healthcare, no mention is made of the potential – positive or negative – of the workplace as another potential source of social support or anguish. This may stem from flawed assumptions that parents, especially mothers, don't work outside the home when they have a child with a chronic illness. Workplaces as a potential avenue of support should be considered.

In this study, insufficient social support was reported, especially reliable social networks that might have been routinely called upon. Social support – from any source – is vital for successful adaptation, coping and survival. Unfortunately, social support for those with disabilities (or their carers) may not always be available, and it may be withdrawn over time. Also, when social support does exist, it may not be supportive or positive (Vickers, 1997a; 2001a).

A lack of support, or a perception of support being absent or unreliable, negatively affects individual and family adjustments to chronic illness and disability. However, little is known about which particular behaviours parents actually perceive to be unsupportive or hurtful (Garwick et al, 1998: 665). It is hoped that what is presented in this chapter will assist. The unsupportive responses of network members that have been studied can be strikingly similar – regardless of the stressful event. Unsupportive behaviours have included: minimising the seriousness of the negative event; forced cheerfulness; avoiding contact with the person; avoiding communication or expression of feelings about the event; criticising or acting judgementally; being overprotective; expressing excessive worry or pessimism; making rude or insensitive comments; and expressing inappropriate expectations about the person's adjustment process (Ingram et al, 2001: 175). Of interest, these kinds of behaviours have been reported for *varying kinds of stressful events* – including one's own chronic illness or disability (Vickers, 2001a), or that of one's child (Ingram et al, 2001). Similarly, no distinction is made here between varying types of illness or disability that the child had. I claim that, as long as an event or situation was stressful to the parent, then Clayton's support made matters worse – regardless of what was wrong with their child.

Unfortunately, Clayton's support was frequently reported in the vivid examples that follow; from:

- Professionals;
- Colleagues;
- Friends;
- Family; and,
- Partners.

Clayton's support: from professionals

We saw in Chapter 1 that the major step of a child entering the school system becomes imbued with issues surrounding the need for the parent to give up control of the child's healthcare management during the day to teachers. Unfortunately, teachers may have little knowledge about the child's chronic illness (Melnyk et al, 2001). Unsupportive behaviours also emanate from other professionals providing support to children with chronic conditions, such as healthcare providers, educators and community members (Garwick et al, 1998: 669–670). Below, Polly described the response from the deputy headmistress at her local school talking about Polly's son, as if Polly was not the caring, loving mother of that child. Unsupportive responses from school providers are frequently observed, with the five most common types being: providing inadequate services; being insensitive to the child's needs; lacking understanding of the child's condition; having inadequate professional knowledge or training; and not recognising the child's problems or needs (Garwick et al, 1998: 670). Unfortunately, all of these were evident in Polly's story. What Garwick and colleagues have not commented on is the Clayton's (unsupportive) response of not recognising the parent's feelings or needs, and being insensitive to them. Polly remembers her dealings with the deputy headmistress at Primary School Y, who demonstrated little, if any, sensitivity to Polly's feelings regarding her son, nor any respect for another parent of a child in the school with a disability (who Polly happened to know):

> **Polly:** Christine's at [Primary School X] for a very specific reason. At [Primary School Y, also located close by], it's 800 kids and they've got a big 'gifted and talented' focus … I went and saw the deputy headmistress … about Thomas going there. This was a long time before he was diagnosed with the leukaemia, and all of the assessments were that he was a number one candidate for mainstreaming. And I thought, 'Fabulous!' She starts to give me the spiel about the high net worth of the families in her school, and how many 'gifted and talented' children there are at the school, and that Thomas would feel all the more '*retarded*' at the school, quote unquote. 'You know, Mrs [Polly's surname], Thomas will feel all the more retarded if he comes to this school'. And I just thought, 'Fuck!' She said, … 'I have the mother of an autistic boy at this school. She's up here every day making a nuisance of herself and, you know, she will

never be able to make that child normal. She can't *make* him normal'.

Researcher: I don't imagine she's trying to.

Polly: The school is legally obliged to take any child that lives in that geographic area ... and I probably just presented to her, not like a mother, as just like a professional, dispassionate person.

Researcher: A corporate person that would understand the 'harsh realities?'

Polly: Yes. So, she completely forgot that I was a mother of a disabled child ... I didn't confront her with it; I just left. But what about a kid that's not gifted and talented? What about little Johnny that wants to grow up to be a shoe repair man, and live a fabulous, constructive life in the community, and be a scoutmaster, and bring value to all the lives he touches? And then I went down to [Primary School X, where her daughter Christine now attends] to see headmistress, with a white hair bun. She said that she would take Thomas, but she was cold to me. I saw her in a room with other parents and she was warm to them, and she sort of turned on the cold and went official. She said, 'Happy to take Thomas. Fine, but you need to work with me, because I will need resources. My only reservation is we would have to assess how he continues at the school if we don't get the level of support that we need'. But professional. She wasn't embracing and, 'I love all Down's syndrome kids' – you never get that – but she was professional. (Polly, Interview 1: 42–43)

There was much present in Polly's text that revealed her experiences with professionals. She shared examples of the first deputy headmistress' behaviour – a senior educational professional working at Primary School Y – as acutely insensitive and unsupportive. Clearly, this woman did not want to take Thomas at that school, and was astonishingly thoughtless and unprofessional in her remarks, not just about Polly's son, but about another mother whose child was at that school. However, I remained surprised that Polly was prepared – seemingly happily – to still accept Primary School X, even though the headmistress there was 'cold' towards her and flagged the possibility that there may be inadequate resources to support Thomas in the future. The school may well have been very good and Polly quite happy, but I heard a school headmistress who was warm and welcoming to the other mothers – presumably with their 'normal' children – and who was cold and pessimistic with Polly. This may be explained by Polly having been grateful to have at least received a professional response, if not a welcoming one.

Sandra also reported her negative experiences dealing with educational professionals who were difficult and unsupportive. The unsupportive behaviour of being insensitive to the child's needs, lacking understanding of the child's condition and not having adequate professional knowledge or training (Melnyk et al, 2001; Garwick et al, 1998) were also all evident in Sandra's reported experiences. Sandra expressed her frustration about school providers and teachers that did not understand her son's condition, ADD, and that, sometimes, their conduct made things worse (for both Sandra and Edward). They also treated Sandra in an insensitive and insulting manner, frequently reducing her (a senior HR professional and executive) to tears:

> **Sandra:** And even now ... we had a situation with Edward where he's basically pretty close to being, the next step and he'll be out. And the teachers have had him on, he's been on 'card systems' all his life, you know, these behaviour modification cards. They put him on a yellow card and at the end of every lesson they have to get a rating and a sign-off. And this kid's had this since he was six years of age. He's been on a card system for the last 18 months at the school, and it's not working. We had this meeting with his housemaster, and I said, 'Can't you see it's not working?' ... But they said, 'This is the way the school does it, and we have to do it this way'. And I said, 'But here's a child that has different needs'. They were going to put him onto a red card system, which basically meant he had a contract to sign. And this red card system, if there was one misdemeanour, it would go before the headmaster and the headmaster would then make a decision as to what action to take; in other words, whether he would stay at the school or not. And I just said to them, 'If you do that to Edward, if you put him onto this now, the anxiety that he has, he will fail' ... So, there's just no flexibility. In saying there's no flexibility, I don't expect him to be treated specially – the same rules apply – but they have to do things a little differently.
>
> **Researcher:** How did *you* feel, when you thought it was going to be one thing and then it was referred to the headmaster?
>
> **Sandra:** I think that it's intimidation and it's harassment. I'd like to take him out of the school, but he doesn't want to. He wants to stay. So we'll support him with that.

Researcher: That's quite a betrayal; that's my reading of the situation.

Sandra: It *is* a betrayal. (Sandra, Interview 2: 4–5)

Unfortunately, different 'psychosocial interpretations' (Meyerson, 1994: 644), different perceptions of illness (Fitzpatrick and Scambler, 1984: 72), and different role expectations (Turner, 1987: 54) may have influenced the professionals' dealings with these women. What Sandra reported may well have stemmed from a lack of understanding of Edward's ADD by the teachers at his school, including their (flawed) perceptions about the nature and seriousness of it, and its impact on his (in)ability to comply with their rules. Sally also reported how draining she found her constant battles with schools and medical professionals, as she battled to get the care she believed her daughter needed. You will recall (see Chapter 3) that Sally felt that it was just 'all too hard' for her to continually do battle with health professionals to get the service her daughter needed. Sally not only had to fight with health professionals, she felt she had to do it with insufficient support from her spouse. (I will return to Sally's perceived lack of support from her partner in the final section of this chapter.) Wendy also reported her tussles with health professionals when they were caring for her daughter. When I asked her what path her child's diagnosis might take in the future, her response led her to describe a situation that took place – in the hospital – that shouldn't have. Wendy's experience of Clayton's support from health professionals was one that at once terrified her daughter and jeopardised her health. Wendy was not impressed:

> **Wendy:** OK. It could shorten her life; it could mean that she has diabetes; it could mean that she develops heart and/or lung problems. It almost certainly means that she'll get progressive muscular weakness starting from the extremities, her father now has it in his shoulders, for example. They say – researchers say – that it affects the personality, the vim and vigour that they have, the self-efficacy; that people can be disinterested, apathetic. It's a neurological disorder, so tiredness, exhaustion, fatigue is a very common thing. It can affect the endocrine system, which is perhaps the explanation for why her parathyroid doesn't work. And when the calcium levels go down, unless they're tested and kept up, she will go into – what's happened once with her – a carpopedal spasm. Do you know about those? [Researcher shakes her head] Firstly the hands start to go like

that [demonstrating her hands going into a very tense, claw-like pose], then the feet; and then what happened to her when she was admitted to hospital – she actually had one in hospital, which is great place to have one, isn't it? – where the whole of her body went rigid, and her heart rate was charging along.

Researcher: Were you there?

Wendy: Yes, I was there.

Researcher: You must have been terrified.

Wendy: *She* was terrified, and I couldn't get the medical staff to really take it seriously. It was triggered by poor medical practice on top of the situation. And that's the kind of thing – when the calcium level drops – but it shouldn't get to that point. (Wendy, Interview 1: 21)

Researcher Note: *Wendy didn't directly comment on her own fear, anxiety or anger here, but I can only imagine that she must have also been terrified and angered. From my own experience with hospitals, my own treatment there, my husband's treatment, my father's serious illness in years past, they are places of great anxiety. If I had witnessed a loved one of mine suddenly spasming the way Wendy described, I would have been terrified and felt very vulnerable and helpless also. I can't help but to project my likely response here, especially when it was my view that Wendy had, again, circumvented talking about her own fears, and her own grief, in this situation.* (Vickers, Researcher Reflections, Thursday, 16 June 2005).

Clayton's support: from colleagues

Hodson (1997) suggested that positive social support *can* exist in the organisational context. However, and unfortunately, Clayton's support was also reported from work associates and the workplace context. The unsupportive actions from other members of the community have been reported elsewhere in the form of insensitive comments, lack of understanding and inadequate support (Garwick et al, 1998: 669). While Garwick and colleagues neglected to discuss workplaces and colleagues, I posit that these same insensitivities and problems of lack of understanding from communities also apply at work. Distressed individuals hide their needs and negative feelings from members of their social network so as not to burden, upset, or scare them off and to ensure that others do not form an impression of them as weak or needy (Silver, Wortman and Crofton, 1990: 400). Nowhere is this more likely to happen than in modern workplaces. We have seen that workplaces can be abusive and intolerant of grief and emotion (see Chapter 4). They are also intolerant of emotions, emotional displays (Hochschild, 1983; Fineman, 1993a; 1993b; 1996; James, 1993; Perrone and Vickers, 2004), and anything that overtly pertains to grief and loss (Vickers, 2005c), or cruelty (Vickers, 2005b). They are a likely context for Clayton's support.

Here, I share Cate's experience of uncertainty and anguish pertaining to her child's slower-than-usual developmental patterns as a result of having autism. Her colleagues were very unsupportive and unhelpful. The picture of Cate's lack of social support was overwhelming. She is speaking here about her employer-sponsored daycare centre that denied her son access. I also remind you that her employer was an organisation that provided support for people with disabilities. Her autistic son was just too much trouble:

> **Cate:** The worst thing was when we had that daycare. The employ-ees were told that this was a daycare that you can use for your kid. And it wasn't here; it was offsite. They said, 'You can use this daycare for your kid, and it's going to be great because you'll get this discount on daycare. And it's inclusionary', meaning they were going to welcome kids with disabilities. It was a regular daycare, with regular kids, but they were targeting others. And I thought that was just awesome. And then when they started it, I said, 'Why don't I send my son to it?' And the person who was running the daycare at the time said that they couldn't handle my son, even though he wasn't even yet two. And they just said that he was too hard to work with for the staff ... And they said, 'No' and I went to them in writing. I said, 'Can you please tell me why you're denying me this, because I don't understand why at the service agency I can't do this'. And the problem, I think, was that the person running the daycare was a financial guy. He was head of the business office at the time. I don't really think he had very much interest in actually helping kids; I think he was interested in the bottom line. And I think he saw numbers and ratios, and he was, 'Well, this kid's just too hard'. But that was the hardest thing. And even that wasn't that big of a deal. It made me grow; it made me branch out into the community for daycare. (Cate, Interview 1: 10–11; Vickers, 2005b)

Supervisors in the workplace can be a great source of stress (Argyle, 1989: 277). Cate's story was reflected in many other respondents' expe-riences, although she was the only one who reported, concurrently, experiencing support withdrawal or absence from her mother, partner, in-laws, colleagues, as well as the employer-sponsored daycare centre.

Clayton's support: from friends

When asked about supportive relationships and friendships, Wendy shared the story of her neighbour's support, making it very clear that she was aware that she could not draw on the support of her neighbour too much. As we saw earlier, the problem of initial support dissipating over time has been recognised elsewhere (Dunkel-Schetter and Bennett, 1990: 278). For Wendy, in addition to her concerns of losing the support she currently had from her neighbour, she felt generally unsupported. This was of grave concern as I could not help but agree with her assessment. Wendy had already reported to me that her estranged husband appeared to only offer emergency assistance, and only when sufficient notice was given so that he would not be inconvenienced (Wendy, Interview 1: 16). Wendy had also confessed that her mother had Alzheimer's and, thus, was not only unable to provide support, but was likely to be another potential source of stress and grief in her life. Wendy described her father as a 'total shit' (Wendy, Interview 1: 15) suggesting that he was not especially supportive either and her elder daughter, who had helped Wendy in the past, as not really having grasped the enormity of the health issues facing Wendy's younger daughter, Samantha. Finally, Wendy's son lived in Canberra (about 300 km from where Wendy lived). She admitted: 'Look, basically, in terms of family support, relatively little; at a distance, and relatively little' (Wendy, Interview 1: 15). Wendy concluded:

> **Wendy:** So, there is a sense of being very unsupported.
> **Researcher:** Yes, I am hearing this.
> **Wendy:** I have a neighbour who's wonderful, who has sort of rushed down the road till I got home and that kind of thing. Who asks, and we see each other every second day probably, and so she's been wonderful. But I've also got to make sure that I don't draw on that friendship, so that the friendship isn't overtaxed or anything. (Wendy, Interview 1: 16)

Sadly, Wendy also reported a situation where two friends she felt very close to had let her down by not staying in contact with her after she had shared her loss and grief over the illness of her daughter. We have seen elsewhere that, while friends may feel helpless, or uncertain as to how to act (Ingram et al, 2001: 174), in this instance, their lack of response (and perceived indifference) served as a major contributor in making Wendy feel even less supported. Avoiding communication with the person, not allowing them to express their feelings about negative events in their lives, and minimising the seriousness of that event (Ingram et al, 2001: 175) all contributed to Wendy's experience of Clayton's support:

> **Researcher:** Are there any other people who you regarded as friends who have disappointed you?
> **Wendy:** Yes. [Laughter] Surprisingly.
> **Researcher:** Can you tell me about it?
> **Wendy:** Oh, I've spoken to two very old friends, you know, the kind of friends you talk to every Pancake Day. And when you do, you're right back there and stuff. And I rang both of them. One was probably three months ago, and the other a couple of months ago. And I haven't heard from them since. And I'm just astounded ... I almost feel like ringing up and saying, 'Did we have a conversation? I know we did'. So, yes.
> **Researcher:** Do you think the whole illness/disability thing's just too scary for them?
> **Wendy:** Look, I don't know. They're people that I have really deep, intimate – not sexual – but really intimate relations with. You know, I'm crying my eyes out on the phone saying, 'I'm going to be in a wheelchair, and she's going to be in a wheelchair'. You know, I have my own fears about Alzheimer's myself ... So I'm somewhat astounded, because I really felt I could count on both of them. (Wendy, Interview 1: 17)

We have seen that members of the social network may not know how to behave or what to do. However, we also know that the most unhelpful and unsupportive (and common) response to people in need is for those around them to avoid contact and to avoid communicating with them about the event or problem (Garwick et al, 1998; Ingram et al, 2001: 175). Wendy was obviously very hurt and surprised by the behaviour of her friends. Sally reported a similarly hurtful example of Clayton's support that happened after the birth of her daughter, Nadine. When Nadine was born and people had heard what was wrong, Sally indicated that they seemed not to know what to do, or how to respond. Sally confessed that the response of her friends after the birth of her baby was as if there had been a death in the family, not a new life:

Sally: There were no gifts, there were no flowers, there was no nothing. It was really interesting. And again, reflecting, I think it was about the Tuesday or the Wednesday, so four, five days later, that my neighbour came in. And she brought a teddy bear and a bunch of flowers. I lie, I got flowers [before her neighbour came in], but no baby presents. That was really interesting. But I guess people don't know what to do. They don't know how to react or what to do. Lots of flowers. It's almost like a mourning kind of –, because I guess that's what people feel comfortable with. Something bad? Send flowers. So my neighbour came with a little teddy bear and I said, 'That's the first baby present I've got!' [imitating a weepy voice]. I started crying again. I thought I'd cried all the tears that I could cry. (Sally, Interview 1: 12)

Clayton's support: from family

Support from spouses, family and friends have been found to have a positive effect on health adaptation among families (Barakat and Linney, 1992; Florian and Findler, 2001; Barnett et al, 2003: 186). Indeed, the positive, protective effects of social support have been well-documented in articles about families who care for children with chronic conditions (Garwick et al, 1998). The size of the family's support system has been noted as the best predictor of lower stress and fewer family difficulties. Unfortunately, there was often a poor match reported between desired and actual family support which had a very negative influence on the lives of respondents.

Family members were often responsible for contributing to the Clayton's support experience. The most common types of unsupportive actions from (extended) family members reported in the literature (and reflected here) included: receiving unasked for advice; having inadequate contact with the child or the child's family; offering inadequate emotional support; lacking understanding about the child's condition; making insensitive or invasive comments; and blaming the parents for the child's condition (Garwick et al, 1998). What was especially troubling was that these women with caring and working responsibilities had a need for social support higher than most. Evalyn reported her bitter upset when a family member, her brother-in-law, would not mind her child so that she could attend church with her family to listen to the sermon. Evalyn had impressed upon me how much her religious faith meant to her. Church attendance with the other members of her family clearly meant a great deal to her. She was weeping quietly after sharing her pain:

Evalyn: Yes! Because I go to church, I found that I couldn't go to church with Kevin, like, listen to a sermon. And I actually, one day, I, I actually had the 'hide' to do a roster for my family; who went to church. And I said, every month, I'd like to be able to sit in with Mathew [her other son], and be a family, and listen to the sermon. And my brother-in-law said, 'We can't do that, because what about our own family? Who's going to look after *our* kids when we're looking after *your* kids?' It was really, he was really negative about it. And I was just devastated. I was absolutely devastated. And then he, after that he actually apologised. [Evalyn became very upset at this point and started to weep.] (Evalyn, Interview 1: 54; Vickers, 2005b)

Evalyn described a common example of Clayton's support from a member of her family. This person, sadly, demonstrated a complete lack of understanding of her needs and also portrayed his inadequate provision of emotional support (Garwick et al, 1998: 669). It was very important for Evalyn to go to church and listen to the sermon with her family and her brother-in-law didn't seem to understand this. When coping strategies fall short and, especially, when a person needing assistance asks for help, it can be devastating for them to learn that the anticipated support is not there, or worse, is actually unhelpful, as her brother-in-law's initial negative response was. Such challenges can detract from marital and family relationships thereby creating further tensions within families (Barnett et al, 2003: 185). Cate shared her experience of Clayton's support when trying to get some child minding support from her mother. Readers will recall that Cate's mother had also raised a disabled son herself (Cate's brother, Brian, who Cate also cared for):

Cate: My mother's 66 ... when I think of her, I look at her and I say, 'You should be able to watch William' – that's his name – 'You should be able to watch Billy no problem because you had Brian'. But she doesn't, and I'm not sure why. I think it's because she's just kind of jaded. I waited a really long time to have kids, and Billy's only four. I'm 38, so that tells you how long I waited [laughter]. And she's 66, and I just think she isn't committed about him. I don't think she wants to deal with it. I think she loves him, but I think it's like, I just can't expect her to come and watch him. Where before I had him, I kind of had this thing in my mind and we talked about it, 'Mum, are you going to be able to help out? Are you going to be able to come over and stay if we want to go out? You know, will you watch the kids?' 'Yes, yes, yes. I'll do that'. But when it came down to it, it's not turning out that way. (Cate, Interview 1: 3; Vickers, 2005b)

When considering social support, what is vital to consider in the first instance is the *perception* of the availability of support, rather than just the amount of support received, and how this perception positively influences psychological functioning in parents of children with chronic conditions (Garwick et al, 1998: 665; emphasis added). Unfortunately, when perceived support isn't met, this has consistently been negatively correlated with measures of distress. If people don't receive the support they expect, or think support is not going to be forthcoming or can't be relied upon, this can be very disturbing.

While it is acknowledged that 'social support is not a bottomless well' (Hobfoll and Stephens, 1990: 465) and that, frequently, people who are potential givers of support may not know how to react when dealing with people during a life crisis (Silver, Wortman and Crofton, 1990: 398), the situation Cate described is different. She had, reasonably, anticipated some support from her mother in terms of childcare based on her discussions and agreements with her mother prior to Billy being born and, I would suggest, because her mother had raised a disabled son herself and would have understood the burden of care required. Having inadequate contact with the child or its parents, or lacking involvement with the child or their family and generally providing inadequate emotional support, are considered to not only be insufficient support, but *unsupportive behaviours* (Garwick et al, 1998: 669). Cate's experience of Clayton's support demonstrated the chasm between expected or anticipated support she had agreed with her mother, and what had transpired. It must have been terribly disappointing and confusing for Cate.

In Chapters 3, 4 and 5, we saw that Cate's colleagues were also not especially supportive. Now, we see that neither her mother nor husband were supportive. People with illness and disability also sometimes have trouble getting the support they require (Silver, Wortman and Crofton, 1990: 397; Vickers, 2001a); these carers of children with chronic illness and disability were similarly troubled. Many members of Cate's social support network depicted inadequate understanding of her child's condition or of her support needs. She appeared to have had enormous difficulty getting *anyone* to help her care for her son. Her solution? Cate *paid* her mother-in-law for assistance:

Cate: I had to go away twice. Once to bring the kids over there so that Colin's Mum could get used to being alone with [Billy]. And then a couple of months later I could actually go and be able to drop [Billy] off there for a couple of days at a time, because she was intimidated by him too. She was, *'What am I going to do with this four-year-old kid who doesn't know how to talk, and still uses a diaper?'* Plus I paid her some money, so that always helps ... they don't have any money, so they were like 'Whoo-hoo!' ... And that's what it took. That's what it took. That's what I had to do. (Cate, Interview 1: 6; my emphasis; Vickers, 2005b)

It is such a difficult time for parents when they learn that their child has a significant, lasting illness or disability. Common parental reactions to the news includes: feeling devastated, overwhelmed and traumatised; shock, denial, numbness and disbelief; feelings of crisis and confusion; loss of the 'hoped for' child; grief reactions; destroyed expectations for the future; feelings of guilt, responsibility and shame; anger; decreased self-esteem and self-efficacy as their sense of self is challenged; marital and other family relationship strains; and the disruption of family routines (Barnett et al, 2003: 188). Having a child with chronic illness sets into motion a number of chronic and acute stress conditions that are likely to detract from the parent's well-being, and the quality of family relationships (Barnett et al, 2003). These women had to endure all this while holding down a full-time job. Dolly shared her experience of Clayton's support, where her mother's provision of well-intentioned support was most unhelpful. She explained:

Researcher: You mentioned about Shelley [Dolly's mother] being quite emotionally demanding. How did that affect you?
Dolly: I didn't realise it did. I don't think I allowed myself to have conscious thoughts about what that was actually doing to my life ... We almost got to the stage where we [Dolly and her ex-husband] were scheduling fights on the weekend [when Dolly's mother wasn't there] ... I also realised, when I was going to counseling – when I was looking at my personal problems this time last year – that I didn't have a defined role with Margaret. He was the player; he was the party-guy; he was the rough-and-tumble fellow; he was a great Dad. And Mum had come in and taken over my job. She bathed, fed, put Margaret to bed – that was her role. If I tried to get in the way of that, she wouldn't let me. (Dolly, Interview 2: 10–11)

Many have confirmed that social support is not *necessarily* supportive or positive (Argyle, 1989: 277; Blaney and Ganellen, 1990: 300; Ray, 1992; Ingram et al, 2001: 174) and those providing support do not always respond in ways that are helpful to one faced with a negative life event. In some cases, even well-intentioned attempts to support may be perceived by the recipient as unhelpful or upsetting (Ingram et al, 2001: 174). Dolly's experience of Clayton's support stemmed from her mother not allowing Dolly to be fully involved with the care of her child.

Clayton's support: from partners

The distinction has been made between available and received support (Dunkel-Schetter and Bennett, 1990: 269), as well as the problem of initial support dissipating over time (Dunkel-Schetter and Bennett, 1990: 278). Support cannot always be relied upon, especially if it is required over long periods as is likely for carers of a child with chronic illness. Supporters may feel vulnerable, helpless, or fearful, or uncertain as to how to act or what to say; or they may hold misconceptions about the nature and duration of the adjustment process (Ingram et al, 2001: 174). These factors may well have played an important role in the stories that follow. Unfortunately, even if such actions were not intended to be harmful, the painful outcomes can be just as real and damaging to careers, lives and families.

Conversely, Bristol and colleagues (1988) found that support from one's spouse was the best predictor of parental quality, a central concern in these women's lives. Support from partners has also been noted to have a positive effect on health adaptation among families (Barakat and Linney, 1992; Florian and Findler, 2001; Barnett et al, 2003), and a good match between actual and desired support has been found to significantly and positively effect personal adaptation to negative life events (Bristol, Gallagher and Schopler, 1988; Garwick et al, 1998; Barnett et al, 2003).

Unfortunately, these women often didn't get spousal support. Cate reported instances of Clayton's support from her partner, Colin. You will recall (see Chapter 2) Cate coming home from work early to find that her partner, Colin, had left both their children (a two-year-old and an intellectually disabled four-year-old) alone in the house. Their father had gone out to purchase more alcohol for himself, leaving both the children home, unsupervised (Cate, Interview 1: 64). Sadly, I share here another example of Colin's unsupportive actions. Cate had confessed that she could not rely on Colin to care for Billy because she was fearful that he might lose control and hurt him. Consequently, Cate had to drop everything at work and return home if her husband needed her to. Cate also avoided leaving their disabled son alone with his father. She shared one situation, though, when she went into hospital to give birth to their second child, where she found it unavoidable to leave Billy with his father. Cate was clearly anxious about what might have happened:

> **Cate:** I'm afraid he'll come out with that some day, he'll try to hurt Billy one day in anger and frustration ... ultimately, I'm not sure if I trust [Colin] alone with him over extended periods of time. So the way I deal with it is that I make sure he [Billy] has care. Meaning, the babysitter is there rather than my husband. And there's never a time when he has to watch that's over three hours. And I am the controller of that; I am the master. That's something I took upon myself ... I mean, he said to me, 'I can't watch these kids. I can't take it; it's too much. Billy's too uncontrollable. He stuck his hand in his diaper and put poo all over the wall. I can't take it'. ... There have been days when he's called me and said, 'Listen, I can't take it. You need to come home *now*'. And I'll go home. And it's rare, but I always make a point – I say to him – '*You* have to call me and tell me before something happens. That is your out. You *need* to call me'. So he understands ... but, like I said, ultimately I don't really trust him alone with him for overnight and stuff like that. Like when I had the second baby, I had to be in hospital overnight, and he was home with Billy, and that was really, really hard ... I asked my mum to stay but she couldn't. But it was fine.
> **Researcher:** Does he know that you have those reservations about his control?
> **Cate:** I don't know. We never talk about it. I never sat down and said, 'I don't trust you'. I just kind of manufacture our schedule so that it doesn't occur. (Cate, Interview 1: 20–21; Vickers, 2005b)

For Cate, not only was support for her in home duties lacking from her partner, her work-life was often interrupted unexpectedly, and she felt unable to leave her disabled child with his own father for any length of time. I would characterise this example of Clayton's support as not only a sharp absence of support, but as a gaping rift between the support one might normally expect from a partner and father of the child, and what could be relied upon. Cate's situation and caring responsibilities appeared overwhelming. While working full-time, she had to care for her son Billy, with autism, her grown brother with a disability, her unsupportive husband, and her able-bodied two-year-old.

Finally, Sally reported her experience of Clayton's support from her partner as ambivalence and exasperation over the years since their daughter, Nadine, had been born. On the one hand, early in the interview, Sally had told me that her partner had been very supportive and really got involved with looking after Nadine, for example, when she needed surgery when she was very young. However, when I sought to confirm this support at a more generalised level, unfortunately, this was Sally's response:

> **Researcher:** So, he's been quite involved in these sorts of things?
>
> **Sally:** Yes and no. Sometimes. Most of the time, I don't know whether he chooses not to be involved or, because I'm so damn assertive and organised and do it, that it's easier for him to take a back seat. It's probably only recently, because she [Nadine] is now getting ready for more cranio-facial reconstructive stuff, that I guess I've sort of said, 'I've been doing it, been fighting these battles for 15 years. It's *your* turn. It's time for *you* to take on some of this stuff'. And maybe that's been part of the driver too for me to move from part-time to full-time [work]. The constant battle, the constant adjudicating arguments. It's almost an escape. I tend to come home now and, while I'm exhausted, I can tune out like he does ...
>
> **Researcher:** Do you wish that Peter had taken more of an active role in those sorts of tussles with the medical fraternity?
>
> **Sally:** Yes, definitely. Because, I think not only to be a support – and it's not that he wasn't supportive – but I think he lacks depth in understanding about what her [Nadine's] issues are, what her difficulties are. Sometimes he'll just go, 'Why can't she do that?' And I'm, 'Because she can't. When are you going to get it? She can't!' (Sally, Interview 1: 18–19)

Needing reliable support

Wendy responded to the presentation of the emergent theme of Clayton's support at the Stage 3, CGE:

> ... like 'Clayton's Support'. I thought, 'Oh yes, I know what that is'! [Laughter] (Wendy, CGE: 10)

Unfortunately, the absence of emotional support and inadequate practical help were common problems (Garwick et al, 1998: 670) reported by the women in this study. Inadequate support was reported in all areas of lives and social networks: from partners; immediate family; extended family; friends; colleagues; as well as educational and health professionals. One possible and hopeful avenue of support that should be explored in the future is reported by Boukydis (1994) who claims that parents of children with disabilities feel that other parents in similar circumstances are those best able to provide the emotional support desired and needed. The most helpful social support for those who have experienced a loss includes contact with those who have experienced similar losses, to share and vent feelings (Barnett et al, 2003: 195). Marital counseling has also been found to have beneficial effects for parents whose child has a medical condition (Barnett et al, 2003: 195). However, few respondents in this study reported undertaking marital counseling; when they did, it tended to be to repair their marriage rather than discuss their child.

Unfortunately, the women in this study had great difficulty accessing the support, formal and informal, that they needed. Because they were working full-time, they simply did not have the time to attend support groups, mother's clubs, and school gatherings (see Chapter 3). Because others were not sensitive to their needs, they often experienced Clayton's support, which made more difficult other issues in their lives, such as grief resolution, coping, family and individual adjustment, relationships, career development, and general well-being. For either formal or informal support to be effective it needs to be positive and reliable – not the Clayton's support witnessed here.

Part III
Enabling Survival

7
Working and Caring

My Husband Ran Over My Son

My husband ran over my son.
Ten months old, a paraplegic
My husband, guilty, couldn't handle my son's disability
We separated.

Pregnant.
My daughter was born, I entered the workforce
No choice, both children
Couldn't handle a full-time job.

Part-time jobs allowed me to come and go
Started a part-time job, a second part-time job
Then, three part-time jobs; 45 to 60 hours a week
We needed the extra money.

I understand –
My husband ran over my son.

(Cate, Interview 1: 1–2, 11)

Revisiting the work-home balance

The need to revisit the challenges surrounding managing work and home has been highlighted (Lewis and Lewis, 1996). As we have already seen, in most parts of the Western world, care for chronically ill children remains mostly the responsibility of mothers (Martin and Nisa, 1996: 3; Burke et al, 1999). Despite the fact that the statistical norm is now for women to work outside the home, cultural beliefs continue to preserve the unequal division of labour in parental care.

Add to this the fact that, over the last two decades, the average worker has added an extra 164 hours – a month of work – to his or her work year and we find both men and, particularly, women overburdened. Workers also now take fewer unpaid leaves, and even fewer paid ones (Hochschild, 1997: 6). While it is acknowledged that, in many cases, men are increasing their daily involvement with home and family, and employers are introducing family-friendly policies designed to assist workers meet conflicting work and home responsibilities, the reports shared here indicated that: (a) these women had a great deal of difficulty combining work and home; and, (b) that the workplace 'flexibility' and support that is so often paraded, may not have been as reliable and dependable as hoped.

What I explore in this chapter are the specifics of these women's workplace experiences and choices in light of their need to balance the demands and responsibilities that guided their lives; namely, their caring and working responsibilities. Examined here are five workplace-related themes that emerged from these women's stories:

- Needing to work;
- Inconstant workplace support;
- Disclosure at work;
- Working and caring; and,
- Work choices.

Needing to work

We know that labour force participation of wives and mothers has increased dramatically during the latter half of the 1900s (Sharpe, Hermsen and Billings, 2002). However, there still remains an expectation in our communities that if a parent, especially a mother, has a child with a significant chronic condition, that the mother will stay home to care for that child. The earlier chapters have confirmed expectations that women, especially mothers, should be selfless, and put the needs of their family ahead of their own on a regular basis – even if it is detrimental to them via increased stress levels, poor health, or missed opportunities. The paucity of literature about full-time working mothers caring for chronically ill children implicitly confirms the widely held view that they should not be working at all, and definitely not working full-time. Respondents confirmed this view. Sally indicated that, after her daughter was born, the expectation from those around her was that she would, simply, devote her life to the needs of her child:

Sally: It was interesting, because afterwards [after the baby was born], I think the expectation was – and not an overt expectation – that I would stay at home to care for this child. [Last words imitating an overly soft, gentle voice] ...

Researcher: People didn't say to you, 'Are you planning to go back to work?' They just didn't ask?

Sally: Probably, yes. They didn't ask; they just assumed that I'd be home now forever to care for this child. (Sally, Interview 1: 14–15)

However, despite the commonplace existence of this assumption, respondents confirmed not only that they did work, but that they *needed to work*; for some, it was not a choice, but a financial necessity. This is confirmed by Kurz (2000: 439) who reports that most mothers want and need to do paid work. Wendy, Dolly, Cate, Charlene and Oitk (all single parents) all reported needing to work to support themselves and their families, and to pay for childcare. Charlene confirmed (in the poem above, and the full text below) that, for 12 long years, she had *three* part-time jobs and worked between 45 and 60 hours per week:

Charlene: I started out with a part-time job. Because I had so many obligations with my son, I couldn't handle a full-time job and both children. And then I ended up with a second part-time job because financially we needed the extra money. And I ended up with three part-time jobs.

Researcher: That was the equivalent of how many hours a week?

Charlene: 45 to 60 hours a week.

Researcher: And you still managed the kids as well with 45 to 60 hours of work.

Charlene: Yes. (Charlene, Interview 1: 2)

While Charlene had a Master of Business Administration (MBA) degree at the time of interview, she was typical of single mothers sucked into the 'bottomless pit of poverty' (Albelda and Tilly, 1998: 43). Single mothers face the same obstacles as other women plus the lack of a spouse's income and support, leaving many of them dependent on government-provided income (Albelda and Tilly, 1998: 43). This is an increasing problem. Fewer and fewer women are getting or staying married. In the US, close to 45 per cent of women are not currently married. Australia is similarly placed: about two-thirds of all first marriages (and an even higher proportion of remarriages) end in separation or divorce (Albelda and Tilly, 1998: 44). Wendy (Interview 1), a divorcee, confirmed that she now needed to continue working to support her daughter for much longer than she originally would have planned. As she approached the latter years of her career, she would normally have been thinking about her options and choices as a woman without dependent children, without a partner, and with the freedom to have chosen other life and career paths. Now, rather than gearing for retirement and a maturing daughter leaving home, she found herself still responsible to care for her daughter. Her teenage daughter had become – with her newly diagnosed chronic illness – a dependent child for much longer than either of them ever anticipated:

> **Wendy:** I guess it means that I need to have an income. I need to think about how to support my daughter when she goes through higher education, and what that means for the kind of living arrangements that she has. And it means that I feel less free to do things that I was trying to gear myself up to do as an empty-nester.
> **Researcher:** What sort of things would you maybe have done if things were different?
> **Wendy:** Well, you see, it leaves me with enormous uncertainty. I think that's the major thing. I don't know whether we'll move to Sydney so that we can both be in the same place, or whether she'll move to Sydney, or whether I'll move to Sydney independently. I can't afford to run two places. Whether I'll stay here, I mean, I would dearly like to just move out of here.
> **Researcher:** Here being your employer?
> **Wendy:** Yes. I would like to leave this employer ... Now I feel like I really will need to take account of her, and that I'd *want* to do that. I really want to do that ... So, I guess the uncertainty, the need to – and the desire to – incorporate her longer than I would have done. And the complexity.
> **Researcher:** Do you have a sense of how much longer you think that might be? Or that's part of the uncertainty?
> **Wendy:** No idea. I can just about work out what we'll do for July [the interview was conducted in June], and that's about how far ahead I think I can go. And I'm finding that really hard. (Wendy, Interview 1: 25)

However, those still in partner relationships also reported needing to work to support families; several respondents indicated that being financially secure enabled choices that made life a lot easier. For example, Sandra confirmed that her considerable earning power enabled her to make choices that assisted with her responsibilities for her son, Edward, through her being able to afford a full-time nanny as her children grew. She was also able to afford to send Edward to boarding school at an exclusive Sydney school, and to counseling when it was needed (Sandra, Interview 1: 11). Sandra made it very clear that without earning the money she did, and having the work flexibility that accompanied working in and managing her own business, life would have been very difficult indeed.

Finally, let us not forget that many of these women *wanted* to be working – for themselves. The development of self is a central part of women's workplace learning. Composing a self and a life through work is often influenced strongly by women's workplaces, even when they are often configured as destructive and divisive economic and social arrangements (Fenwick, 1998: 199). For many of the women in this study, meaning making and the development of self, happened when some aspect of their experience or self was challenged (Fenwick, 1998: 200). These women created meaning from their workplace experiences – good and bad – so that they could continue to peel away layers to discover their core, essential, authentic self, while also creating moment-by-moment new dimensions and perspectives of self (Fenwick, 1998: 201). This was Sally's reason for returning to work and why Oitk continued studying for her degree, with some difficulty at times – to do something for themselves. Polly confirmed her expectation that after Thomas was born she would return to work, as before. Work, in and of itself, can be of great value to individuals, families and societies. For individuals, it may be a source of pride, self-fulfilment, and social contacts, and it may enhance time structure. For families and societies it can provide a mechanism for providing food, shelter and other services (Gjerdingen et al, 2000: 2). While Polly subsequently reflected that her return to work full-time might not have been very sensible, it was her choice to make:

Researcher: Right, and then Thomas was born. And I imagine when Thomas was born, as you said, they [her former employer] mapped out the path for you: 'Be at this place, do these things'.
Polly: But [former employer] was fabulous, and my boss was fabulous. Mapped out the path, my job was always there for me after the birth and the assumption was that I would return sort of immediately. And we never discussed part-time. And I don't know what I was thinking I was going to do. But we had a place booked ... and

they had a nursery, with all these babes in arms, and here was Thomas just going to go into the nursery, and it was just going to be this fabulous fast-lane life, you know, that everyone does. Because I was an absolute sucker for the propaganda of the feminist movement from the early seventies.

Researcher: Yes. 'You can have it all'.

Polly: 'You can have it all'. And until you do it, you've got no idea. (Polly, Interview 1: 7–8)

Of course, Hewlett (2002: 66) exposed the myth of executive women 'having it all', making it clear that, for many women, the brutal demands of ambitious careers, the asymmetries of male-female relationships, and the difficulties of bearing children late in life conspire against women. She also pointed to the heavy costs involved (Hewlett, 2002). What was interesting in Polly's comments was that, while she exercised her right to return to full-time work in a senior executive position, there was cynicism evident as to how she thought, at the time, it would all be very easy: that life would just carry on; that having her son with Down's syndrome was just a bump in the road. However, while she learned that working full-time and caring for her child was not so easy, it was still her right. What I saw were women coming to know and appreciate their power and performance, sometimes with success and inner resources that surprised them. Like the women in Fenwick's study, as these women came to feel their power, they became more confident and learned to trust their own voices (Fenwick, 1998: 203).

Inconstant workplace support

One of the primary objectives in this study was to learn how respondents lived the crossover between work and home, especially given their additional caring responsibilities. The concept of the workplace being hostile, abusive or sick is not new (see Chapters 4 and 5) and is closely linked with managerialist and capitalist doctrines. Managers have long been reported to be inconsiderate of staff, either as a result of ignorance, thoughtlessness, power and politics, or the pursuit of unreasonable efficiency objectives. Workplaces are sources of feelings of isolation, powerlessness and alienation.

The recent recognition of workplace abuse and aggression, bullying, psychological abuse, workplace incivility and aggression, points to an increasingly challenging arena for parents trying to balance work and family. Phenomena such as downsizing, restructuring, and an increased emphasis on lean and mean organisations continues to place pressure on workers to spend longer hours, perform at a higher level, and be fearful for their jobs.

Knowing this, I braced myself for ugly stories of victimisation, unfair dismissal, discrimination, alienation, lack of understanding, and general brutishness from managers, employers and colleagues. While glimpses of such events were reported, they were neither universal nor common. Instead, the stories provided a very mixed response to the question of workplace support (Vickers, 2005d). We should certainly not assume that all is well. When respondents did indicate supportive colleagues and work environments, they *always* tempered these comments, making it clear that they believed their positive workplace experiences were not routine, nor to be expected elsewhere. Those reporting positive workplace experiences appeared *grateful* to find themselves so placed. However, many provided ambivalent reports, demonstrating their assumptions about the whimsical nature of workplace support and how peculiar circumstances had contributed, in their view, to the positive outcomes they experienced.

Some reported very supportive workplaces, sometimes over lengthy periods of time. For example, Oitk spoke of support from her colleagues, enabling her to swap her workdays at short notice, enabling her to continue her part-time studies. Sandra, Polly and Dolly shared strong sentiments as to support received from their colleagues, and Evalyn also portrayed experiences of understanding and accommodation from her current colleagues and managers, especially as this pertained to her need for flexibility at work:

> **Evalyn:** And so, my managers here, Peter and Rowena, they are just really wonderful and they've been very accommodating and they've ... been extremely supportive about me working at home and that sort of thing. I mean, I'll give you an example. I had a really good friend who was my boss. This was at, I used to work for, at [name of previous employer, a bank]. I mean he used to complain when I went and took time off to see my gynecologist when I was pregnant. You know, and I just said, 'I can't help it! I've got to go. It's every month I have to go, every month or every six weeks I have to go. There's nothing I can do.' And he would let me go but it was just coming to work you just felt you have to go through the whole thing again.

Researcher: Have there been any negative situations pertaining to Kevin?
Evalyn: No, no. No. There really hasn't been. I've been extremely fortunate. You know, but I have to say he's never been that sick while I've worked here. (Evalyn, Interview 1: 30–33)

Ambivalence resonated in Evalyn's account. First, Evalyn pointed out that Kevin had not been acutely ill while she had worked at her current job, confirming her uncertainty as to how a return of her child's acute illness, necessitating increased interruptions to her work, might be received. She also, notably, recounted her experiences with a less supportive workplace elsewhere. In an earlier job – where she worked before she had Kevin – Evalyn reported her manager making her feel uncomfortable about attending medical appointments during her pregnancy. These experiences with a manager who was not supportive of her needs may well have contributed to her concerns pertaining to her current employer. Evalyn also emphasised how fortunate she was in her current workplace, indicating her concern that this might change. She also confirmed her belief that the support she received from her current employer was related to her being employed in the public (versus private) sector (Interview 1). She commented on the family-friendly and flexible workplace practices in that environment and believed that, in the private sector, she would not have been so fortunate. Polly (Interview 1) confirmed the same sentiment with regard to her more recent work choices in the public sector.

Evalyn also described her experiences in another workplace where she had worked and felt supported; an organisation that provided disability support services. She believed this was the reason for their generosity. Cate echoed a similar experience, reporting a positive work environment in the same kind of organisation. Cate reported the understanding of her boss, who had a disabled daughter, and added that a member of the board of directors also had a child with autism (Cate, Interview 1: 25). That these senior managers understood her circumstances, better than most, was clearly a plus. Cate also reported one of her disabled clients offering her money to assist with her childcare costs. She was most appreciative:

Cate: Yes, definitely, including a man who's a consumer of services here offering family support – money – to me to pay for childcare ... Because you would think that it would be a conflict of interest. But it's a program that tries to encourage inclusion of kids with disabilities in summer camp. So they let ... that happen. So it was like, 'Cool'. (Cate, Interview 1: 10)

However, Cate was also very aware of how things might have been different for her elsewhere. She had (see Chapters 3 and 6) also reported profound difficulties working at this same organisation, when seeking care for her child in the organisation-sponsored daycare centre. Cate appeared to have been discriminated against by her employer on this occasion, because of her child's disability. Powell (1998: 95) described the abusive workplace as a workplace that operates with callous disregard for its employees, not even displaying what might be considered a minimum amount of concern for the human needs of staff. That kind of rampant disregard was manifest when Cate was unable to get her child into the daycare centre. So, while Cate's workplace experiences were sometimes positive, they were tempered with events that indicated a complete and callous disregard for her needs – and from those who should have known better.

Other respondents who described supportive workplaces also confirmed their belief that their experience was not universal. For instance, Sandra believed that the reason she received support where she worked was because she was 'the boss'. Similarly, while Dolly reported support at her workplace when her daughter first became ill, she also emphasised that, at the time, she had been the human resources director and responsible for the family-friendly policies underpinning the support she received. She recalled:

Researcher: Did you tell them when you were at [a large corporation] about the problems you were having with Maggie?
Dolly: Yes. They were great.
Researcher: Were they?
Dolly: Extraordinarily supportive, absolutely. Yes, very family-friendly. Well, you know, the irony here is that I was the HR director so I *wrote* the family policies; I *wrote* the maternity leave policies. So I took advantage of it. You know, I *wrote* the telecommuting policy. So, I had other people that I worked with, obviously senior colleagues and that, but they were all extraordinarily 'Just do whatever you need to do'. I mean, I'd put in five and a half-years of extraordinarily hard work, ... energy and effort into helping them grow this business, so they were not at all shy about payback. We had a sick leave policy which ... was unlimited. So, if I wanted to

just go off and not come back for long periods of time, I could have done that. (Dolly, Interview 1: 9)

Workplace entitlements are important. Entitlements such as parental leave and flexible work hours play an important role in mediating between two, often competing institutions – work and family (Baxter, 2000: 13). The availability of leave and flexible work arrangements, as well as favourable attitudes toward these entitlements on the part of employers and coworkers, is important. Dolly also confirmed the uniqueness of the support she received, with colleagues having gone beyond the requirements of policy. They had been personally very supportive – not just because they 'had to be':

> **Researcher:** Were there any examples of colleagues that you worked with at the time that were *particularly* helpful or supportive?
> **Dolly:** My own team was. And two of my directors that I actually worked with ... were particularly –, I was also probably particularly close to them too. They were kind of like 'father figures' to me in some ways, and quite nurturing. One had five children of his own and, you know, his wife's a nurse, so she was obviously actively interested and always calling up, finding out how she was going and things like that. Yes. (Dolly, Interview 1: 9–10)

Wendy also spoke of support at her workplace, but also shared her ambivalence towards the support she had received. Initially, Wendy told me that her immediate colleagues were very supportive:

> **Wendy:** I'd have to say that the people in [name of Department] ... have been nothing other than supportive. They've been really good. I had to change my first night of teaching because she was sick. And I had to change a seminar ... because she was very sick. On both occasions, I just notified them as a professional informing my colleagues. (Wendy, Interview 1: 6–7)

However, concurrent with the understanding she received from some, Wendy had also experienced unanticipated changes in the actions of some of her colleagues that clearly puzzled her, and that she felt were not helpful at all:

> **Wendy:** There are other members of staff who I think, perhaps, might have felt a need to take a step back in case they became 'the

counselor' or something like that ... And that's actually been quite hard, because I would never have positioned them as 'the counselor' ... I noticed we'd always say, 'How's your weekend?' 'Oh, it's been shit. I've been up with sick kids'. And all that [professional] banter has disappeared. And I feel quite uncomfortable with that. In fact, I even do it deliberately now. I sort of say, 'Oh, Samantha's really well this week' or something like, 'How's your kid?' so as to sort of say, 'Well, I haven't silenced myself. You might have silenced me about my kid'. But yes. So, there's been some redefining, both positive and losses ... And then there's been other people, like [name of another colleague], for example, who has been through his own challenging health situations in his family, who has said, 'How's your daughter, Wendy? Have you got some support?' or 'I noticed you were quite upset when I asked you. Are you OK?' So, that sense of not over doing it, but just that human stuff, without having to do counseling or be a counselor or feel like –
Researcher: Just being concerned?
Wendy: Yes. So it's been a range of things. (Wendy, Interview 1: 8–9)

Again, we see that certain individuals were very considerate and thoughtful, while others distanced themselves – and contributed to silencing her, consciously or unconsciously (see Chapter 3). Wendy also shared her belief that her managers, in particular, were most unhelpful. So, while Wendy started the conversation with commentary about colleagues being very supportive, as the discussion continued, a very unpleasant picture began to surface. What troubled me greatly in the following narrative, was that information about Wendy's 'situation' had been passed up the chain, without her consent or knowledge. While I am open about my own chronic illness, I am acutely aware that others are not, and Wendy had impressed upon me that she was very protective of her daughter's privacy. I was, initially, surprised that this event seemed not to have provoked her anger. However, the other appalling behaviour of her manager was probably occupying her thoughts at the time:

Wendy: [Senior manager] was made aware by the [line manager] ... who was trying to do it all 'right' [meaning 'by the book'], of my daughter being ill. You know, I was sometimes working from home ... or whatever.

Researcher: How did you feel when he told [senior manager]? Because you hadn't asked him to, I gather?

Wendy: No, I hadn't asked him to or not. It didn't worry me particularly, but it's more really a style of his management which is more appropriate to 1920s industrialism ... little diagrams on the board telling me how I'd been behaving ... But, I mean, there's also a tremendous amount of patronising in it as well: 'I'm ringing to let you know, [line manager], that I need to put the seminar off. Samantha is not well. Is that fine by you?' ... You know, paying the courtesy. But, at the same time, the response that comes back [from line manager]: 'Well, now tell me, Wendy. *If* you were to go, *how* would you manage? Would you have your mind on the job or would you have your mind at home?' And I said, 'Oh well, of course I'd have my mind at home'. '*Well*, you just answered my question, haven't you? Of course, it's all right ... It's better for you; it's better for your daughter; and it's better for [others involved]'. [Wendy mimics a patronising tone of voice.] So, it's like this kind of benevolent, pompous ass.

Researcher: Patriarchy really, isn't it?

Wendy: It's really pompous! But that's the way that he's managing it. (Wendy, Interview 1: 8)

Interestingly, in the next section it becomes clear that Wendy was indeed incensed by her colleague disclosing personal information about her daughter's illness without Wendy's permission. I turn now to another area of ambivalence and adaptation, especially at work: the question of disclosure.

Disclosure at work

When a man [*sic*] discloses his experience to another, fully, spontaneously, and honestly, then the mystery that he was decreases enormously. When a man discloses himself to me, my preconceptions about him are altered by the facts as they come forth – unless, of course, I have a vested interest in continuing to believe untruths about him. (Jourard, 1971: 5)

Research has shown that persons will permit themselves to be known when they believe their audience has good intentions. Self-disclosure shows an attitude of love and trust (Jourard, 1971: 5). Unfortunately, the disclosure of truth, the truth of one's being, is often penalised. Nowhere might this be more anticipated than in one's place of work. Self-disclosure requires courage, not just the courage to be the person one is, but also the courage to be known by others as one knows oneself to be (Jourard, 1971: 6–7). So, why might a child's illness be a possible source of nondisclosure, especially at work? How might parents feel about telling other people about their child's condition?

Illness can have a profound psychological impact on the individual (Vickers, 1997a; Vickers, 2001a) with psychological responses varying depending on the individual personality, cultural milieu and the illness (Vickers, 2001a). How individuals react to illness also depends on their perceptions of themselves, their body images, and how they feel significant others and society views them (Mead, 1955; cited in Lambert and Lambert, 1979: 2). These same factors are relevant when considering the response to and disclosure of a serious chronic illness in one's child. The presence of disease (with or without symptoms) may invoke a change in the personal identity of the bearer (Fabrega, 1981: 511), and raise concerns for the parent as to how best to address this new identity 'additive' in their child. Illness or disability can over-shadow the individual's personal identity; impairment in Western society is considered the 'worst thing' that can happen to a person (Susman, 1994: 19; Vickers, 2000). Issues surrounding a child's chronic illness are bound to arise for parents too.

Concerns for working parents may relate to the perception that others may have of them – especially at work – as to their capacity to fulfil their work responsibilities. Social and managerialist pressures encourage nondisclosure of a child's chronic illness, especially in the work context. Of interest is the paradox that Jourard (1971: 6) observed regarding the disclosure of anything that may be perceived negatively by others. Jourard (1971) explained the Western *expectation* of disclo-sure and yet the penalty upon doing so: 'Impossible concepts of how man [*sic*] ought to be – which are often handed down from the pulpit – make man so ashamed of his true being [or their child's true being] that he [*sic*] feels obliged to seem different, if for no other reason than to protect his [or her] job'. The penalty that Jourard is referring to is *enacted stigma* (Scambler, 1984: 215) (or discrimination) (Vickers, 1997a; 1997b; 2000; 2001a). Enacted stigma has two perspectives: the socially determined and the personally accepted. Stigma is not just the outcome of other people's devaluations of differentness. For stigma to exist, individuals possessing the differentness must also accept this devaluation (Jacoby, 1994: 269; Vickers, 1997b; 2000; 2001a).

Several respondents demonstrated concern about telling colleagues about their child's condition (Sally, Polly, Sandra, and Wendy). This may have been out of concern for themselves and their careers, concerns for their child – or both. As noted in the previous section, Wendy's manager passed personal information about herself and her daughter's illness to a senior manager, without consulting her. When I asked her about it, at the time, she seemed unconcerned. However, she returned to this question in the next interview – with some determination. She had obviously reflected on this between the first and second interviews. I asked her for some clarification about who she wasn't telling about her daughter's diagnosis, and why:

> **Researcher:** So, you're not going to tell any of your colleagues about her diagnosis?
> **Wendy:** No.
> **Researcher:** Can you tell me exactly why?
> **Wendy:** I've told only one, who's a very close friend; who's a colleague who's become like a friend. And why? [sigh; pause] I don't think it serves to have a label. I think if –, part of it is coming from Samantha not wanting to label herself, it's partly respecting that ... Secondly, because it's not an obvious situation, so it's something that doesn't necessarily need to be named. And thirdly, I guess there's something about protecting my own privacy. A warning from you, an experience myself of saying something and it being repeated, and not wanting to have to explain because the disease isn't understood, it's not in the community as well. All of that. (Wendy, Interview 2: 3–4)

Wendy, like Sandra, did not want her child labeled by her illness. Also represented in her response was the choice that accompanies unseen chronic illness (Vickers, 2001a), especially as it pertained to the employment context – the choice of disclosure (Vickers, 1997a: 240; 2000; 2001a: 81). Self-disclosure of illness or any other potentially stigmatising trait (Jourard, 1971: 6; Vickers, 2000) is a major and complex decision. In this example, not only was Wendy's daughter needing to make choices of disclosure for her own complex reasons, so was Wendy. The information game (Goffman, 1969: 7) and the choice of information control (Goffman, 1963: 113; 1969: 123) rested with these mothers. Even if their child had a chronic illness that was visible, because the child was not usually present in the workplace, the parent still retained a choice regarding disclosure of the child's condition. I also link this to the self-presentation dilemma that exists for people in crisis; whether to present positively, negatively, or portray a balanced coping ability (Silver, Wortman and Crofton, 1990: 402–405) to encourage support from those around them. Disclosure of a child's illness is a complex and challenging question, especially when considered in the work world:

> To display or not to display; to tell or not to tell; to let on or not to let on; to lie or not to lie; and, in each case, to whom, how, when and where. (Goffman, 1963: 57)

Sally captured the essence of the self-presentation dilemma when talking about her decision regarding disclosure of her daughter, Nadine's, condition to colleagues at work.

Researcher: Where you're working now, do they know about Nadine's difficulties?
Sally: The staff, do you mean?
Researcher: Yes.
Sally: Only some people, not everybody.
Researcher: What influences your decision about who you tell?
Sally: I think initially, when I first started working at the [name of hospital], I didn't tell people because I wanted – not so much about keeping my personal life from my private life – but I felt that I needed to establish my credibility as a professional first before I started. Because I don't have a problem in telling people, but I just felt that sometimes it's about timing and about situations. Sometimes it's appropriate, and sometimes it's just not.
Researcher: What about when you applied for the job, and did the interview and all of that, did you tell anyone then?
Sally: No. No.
Researcher: Any particular reason?
Sally: Again it was probably about timing and situations. I don't think it's appropriate; I don't think it's anyone's business at interview. No, not at all. (Sally, Interview 1: 5–6)

Below I have included one of the vignettes that addressed the question of disclosure, based in large part, on Sally's expressed views.[1] Vignette 5 (Part II) spotlit some of the concerns and discomfort that surrounded disclosure issues for these women, especially in the workplace. The vignette was designed to draw attention to the possibility that their child's illness might have been perceived as a 'career-block' – by themselves or by others:

Vignette 5: Feeling different, alone
Part II

At your work there is a big annual, staff barbeque coming up. All the families and children are invited. Everyone is going to be there, even senior management. You are coming up for promotion very soon, and have been encouraged strongly by senior staff to apply and publicly praised for your recent achievements.
Does senior management know about your child? Will you take your child to the barbeque? (Vignette 5, see Appendix)

Not all respondents who received this vignette were concerned about disclosing their child's illness at their place of work. Evalyn reported being completely open about her child's illness, and had portrayed a supportive environment in her current workplace. She showed no sense of felt stigma attached to her child's condition:

> **Evalyn:** Now that's interesting, that's very, very interesting. [Long pause] Firstly, senior management know about my child. In my current situation, senior management does know about my child … I'd have to know what kind of environment that it [the barbeque] is going to be. If it's around a big pool where there's no fencing or anything, then there's no way I'd take my child because it would be a *totally* stressful situation for me. I'd be constantly worried about my child jumping into the pool. So, that kind of thing, I wouldn't. But if it was out in a big park somewhere, and if my husband was going – *if I had adequate support* – I'd take my whole family, because that's my family. And I happen to think my children are very attractive [laughs]! And even if Kevin was slightly different looking or something, that's life nowadays. I mean, Kevin goes to a regular school, with a high support unit attached to it. So … he's no different. I mean, even if he was different, he's no different, if you know what I mean. (Evalyn, Interview 2: 13; emphasis added)

However, other respondents were very much more concerned about the disclosure of their child's condition, for various reasons. For example, Sandra (Interview 1) reported that her son, Edward, was very sensitive about having ADD and she was careful to respect that. She also reported not wanting to let anyone know of some of Edward's more notable temper outbursts and difficulties with anger management. She did not, for instance, want anyone to know about an incident where Edward became very angry – out of control – and threatened members of his family with a knife. Similarly, Sally and Wendy chose not to tell their colleagues about their child. Sally recalled:

> **Sally:** I'm probably a bit naughty sometimes, because I probably use it, not as a shock thing; that's really mean. But I guess people, society in general, devalues people with a disability and, as health professionals, we are members of society. And tragically I think it's reflected in the work that we do as nurses. So sometimes I'll find myself in situations where they'll be having a really derogatory conversation around, you know ... 'Did you see that ... [disabled] kid out in bed eight?' And I just cringe. So I might say things like, 'That's probably somebody's daughter. It could be my daughter, you don't know that'. 'Oh yes, Sally, right'. [being sarcastic]. 'Well actually, I have a daughter with a disability'.
> **Researcher:** Good for you! What happens then?
> **Sally:** 'Ohhhh –,' People aren't freaked out about it, but I sort of use it to put people back in their box. 'Be warned. You just never know who around you has a child with a disability'. Generally people, I don't feel that they go, 'Ugh' [indicating dislike or disgust]. I think it gives them another perspective of who I am and where I'm coming from. Perhaps it gives them a better insight into what I'm all about. (Sally, Interview 1: 9)

When Sally chose to disclose her daughter's disability, she revealed a great deal about herself, that others would not have known. She was revealing some of her mystery, allowing others to know her more. Wendy also spoke of difficulty talking to people about her daughter's illness. She felt unsure what to say, and to whom, when, where and how:

> **Wendy:** One time talking to [name of colleague], and he said, 'Oh, I'm terribly sorry to hear about your daughter'. And it was like it hit me out of nowhere, because I wasn't expecting it. And when I thought about it afterwards, I must have said something to [name of colleague] at some stage. But it hit me out of nowhere ... And what I did, I cut him right off and I totally ignored it, and I went straight

on with the business of the day. And I was absolutely stunned at what I'd done ... And what he was doing was really quite nice actually, but it caught me off guard, and I just went whoosh, straight to the bit of work. And that was quite a strange experience.
Researcher: You were surprised at your own response? Do you think it was because you didn't want to go into that emotional realm with him?
Wendy: I think so. I think so.
Researcher: Too much going on, and you didn't want to talk about it?
Wendy: Yes. And in fact, you asked me why didn't I want to tell people, that's right. [Pause] ... I think because ... the most important thing for me in managing all this is Samantha's self-efficacy ... She said, 'I'd like to be able to forget all about it and get on with my life' ... 'I don't want to be a hero and I don't want to be a victim; I want to get on with having a normal life'. She sees herself, irrespective of the illness, as a pretty normal, average person. And so I think I didn't want her constructed – by others' goodwill or not goodwill – as anything other than that. But I'm still finding it quite difficult to come to terms with how I'm going to do that in the practicality. (Wendy, Interview 1: 27–28)

The difficulties surrounding self-disclosure are significant. We have known for some time that these difficulties frequently associate with stigmatising conditions, such as disability or illness, and may present problems for people in a work context (Vickers, 1997b; 2000; 2001a). However, here were even more complex contexts for disclosure choices. First, these women needed and wanted to acknowledge and respect their child's choice of disclosure, especially if it might have entailed any kind of pigeonholing of their child that might have been harmful, now or in the future. Second, they needed to give thought to their own situation. Whether their choices surrounding disclosure were made consciously, or unconsciously, issues that might have been influential could have included: whether they believed their child's disability was stigmatising for them; whether knowledge of their child's disability might have disadvantaged them, especially at work, such as when being considered for more senior roles, or jobs entailing long hours or lots of travel; whether they trusted those around them sufficiently to share such intimate information, especially in a work context; and, whether they cared what those around them thought. Few with stigmatising conditions will willingly disclose their existence

(Jourard, 1971; Vickers, 2000; 2001a), especially if they believe it will harm them or those close to them.

Unfortunately, their choice of disclosure at work may have vanished during a child's acute illness episode, urgent hospitalisation or lengthy diagnostic journey. As with working adults with chronic illness, the journey to diagnosis is often undertaken by one naïve to the stigmatising nature of illness and disability; respondents may have been 'disclosure ignorant' (Vickers, 1997b; 2000; 2001a: 83). The journey to their child's diagnosis may have been characterised by frustration, grief and loss which may have been shared with colleagues at work along the way (Vickers, 1998; 2001a). The temporal dimension is critical and crucial to our understanding of being (Mackie, 1985: 75). Work absences and sick leave need to be explained. People who learn of their child's serious illness over the phone while at work are unlikely, at such a stressful time, to carefully consider the ramifications of their disclosure choices at this time (Vickers, 2000; 2001a). Until parents have experienced the consequences of stigma, especially as it relates to them or their child, they may be naïve to its deleterious consequences.

Working and caring

One of the first areas of difficulty for women working and caring was, if during their working day, something happened to their child. Their child might have been at school, or at home with a carer, or in a daycare centre. But if something happened, for example, the child became unwell or was misbehaving, it was the mother who was called to respond. Wendy, Sandra, Dolly and Evalyn all reported the 'awful feeling' they experienced when the phone rang at work to inform them of a problem with their child. Wendy, in particular, discussed the stress this caused for her, describing her heart racing and real anxiety being experienced (see also Chapter 4). She shared a typical situation:

Wendy: There have been a number of occasions where, one, I've had a specialist appointment that I've needed to take my daughter to. I've let them know in advance that I wouldn't be there, and that's been fine. Another occasion where she was ill and I needed to stay with her – that was fine too. It was just, 'Wendy's daughter's not well' to the [line manager]. And where I've been rushing off because I've suddenly got a phone call, then that's been fine. There's been times when I've said … 'I need to have my mobile on at the moment. I may not get a call but I need to have it on because of a family illness'. The problem is, when it rings my heart goes *aah, aah, aah* ... But the impact of that is that when I ring my daughter, or when she rings me, there's always this sense of: *'Oh shit!'* [expressing great concern].

Researcher: What's happening now?

Wendy: Yes, yes. Mostly it's not a big deal, but there was a short period of crisis with heart palpitations and she was very scared and there was stuff going on. It was the unpredictable nature of the illness. It's not as though, OK, she's got the flu; you stay at home and take leave. (Wendy, Interview 1: 7; Vickers, 2005c: 211)

The often unpredictable nature of their situations meant that these women felt 'on a knife's edge'. Cate was often called to the childcare centre to attend to her son:

Researcher: Have you ever been called away from work to go to the daycare to attend to him?

Cate: Yes, uh-huh.

Researcher: Often?

Cate: Not too often. In the beginning, more often than now. Every once in a while now. Because if he's sick, you know, they have their rules about picking them up if he's been sick at the daycare ... and they can't really handle him. I go over there and help with it. (Cate, Interview 1: 2)

However, Cate also reported feeling increasingly uncomfortable about doing this, especially what her staff might think about her repeated tardiness:

Researcher: What's been the response of colleagues when you've asked for time off?

Cate: Just fine. My supervisor says, 'Do it. Go ahead' ... There's never been a problem. Not yet.

Researcher: You make up the time or, how do you deal with it?

Cate: I just use sick time. You see, I just get a salary. I don't have hourly [pay]. So, if it's a scheduled time off, I can ask for it. I have a ton of vacation time. I don't usually take it. But he'll just give me the time. I can make it up if I want. Usually he doesn't make me ...

Researcher: Do you feel that others think you're taking too much time off?

Cate: Sometimes I do, yes. Like, if I say, 'I've got to go'. This is the thing, because I'm the supervisor, there's lots of times in the morning when I drop off my son to the daycare ... when I drop him off at the daycare, I have to stay there because the morning time is hard. Either because the staff don't know what to do with him or he goes off about something or there's a new staff member who has no clue how to work with him. And I have to sit down with her and talk with her about it ... But I have to stay, I'll have to come in a little bit late. And then everyone who works here will see me come in late. Then I have to go and find the person who came in late that day and counsel *them* on coming in late when I don't provide a good example myself. And not everybody knows what I'm doing because I have 30 people. How are they all going to know? So, that's one thing. (Cate, Interview 1: 11–12)

Cate was talking about her reaction to being delayed at the childcare centre, either to settle her son down for the day or to liaise with the childcare workers. Cate, as a supervisor of others, then faced the task of admonishing her staff when *they* were late, despite being late herself. Cate felt discomforted by the double standard and worried what her staff might have been thinking. Another area of work-related restriction Cate worried about was her inability to move from where she currently lived. She reported her complete dependence upon her carefully constructed support network:

Researcher: Does having William mean you're restricted to working here in [city where she lives], or do you feel you're able to be mobile still if you want to take a job, for example, back in [a place miles away]?
Cate: *No way.* That's one of the big things why we're still here, for me. Once again, we don't talk about this. We talk about, if we moved, we could actually play out with our band and we could do a lot of things. But the family wouldn't, I'd lose the connections I have. I wouldn't have the same connections I have. And I just told Colin, 'You need to wait'. I need to wait until William is stable. I need to see where he is going with all this autism stuff. (Cate, Interview 1: 25)

Cate is referring to one of the most serious issues that arose for these women; their difficulty finding carers for their child. They had more difficulty than most finding carers because, often, their child required more or different care, and needed it for longer periods. A child with special needs may continue to need care, all day, with this need continuing well into adulthood. Carers may also need to be especially patient, knowledgeable and skilled (see Chapter 3). Cate, for example, had found herself cut off from many of the traditional areas of support available to parents, such as friends and family, other mothers at the local school, or mother's club gatherings. Cate had many of these choices closed to her because of her full-time work. She had no time to network with other mothers, and the pool of potential carers – family members, friends, local teenagers, or professional carers – was restricted by the special needs of her child.

Finally, working and caring entailed taking time away from the workplace to tend to the child, especially during acute illness phases. For Charlene, having several low paid jobs was the only way she was able to find the flexibility she needed to care for her son:

> **Charlene:** There were doctor visits.
> **Researcher:** Very frequent?
> **Charlene:** Yes. I could almost count on him having pneumonia twice a year, at the season changes … He'd be in hospital for a week with pneumonia.
> **Researcher:** Right, still very small then, so you'd have to spend a fair bit of time at the hospital?
> **Charlene:** I'd have to spend a fair bit of time at the hospital. Plus, at that time he was going through evaluations, and therapy and that type of thing too.
> **Researcher:** So there was a fair bit of extra load on you … How did you deal with it? For example, if he's sick for a week with pneumonia twice a year, what happened with your bosses at work? How did that work out?
> **Charlene:** I had low-paying jobs with no benefits, minimum wage, and they were part-time. And they were accommodating to me in that the reason I had those jobs was because I could have time off. I could work the schedule around him.
> **Researcher:** Were you paid on an hourly rate?
> **Charlene:** I was paid on an hourly rate.
> **Researcher:** So you could just adjust your shifts? …
> **Charlene:** I did that because I didn't think I would be able to take a full-time job with an employer and have the flexibility and the time I needed with my son. I didn't visualise any employer hiring me on a full-time basis and letting me have the time off I would need.
> (Charlene, Interview 1: 3)

In Australia, approximately 43 per cent of women in the labour force are in their childbearing years, a significant change from past decades (Baxter, 2000: 13). If both men and women have access to flexible work hours and parental leave entitlements, there will be fewer structural features within workplaces that support traditional gender divisions of labour. A range of workplace policies have been introduced in Australia in recent years – such as parental leave and flexibility in work hours – which have been designed to offset the impact of gender on the division of labour in the home (Baxter, 2000: 13). When children are sick or require treatment, parents must further divide their time between normal responsibilities and caring for their hospitalised child (Melnyk et al, 2001). For Charlene, multiple part-time jobs allowed her to pay the bills and care for her child.

Work choices

The increased involvement of women at work was called a 'subtle revolution' (Smith, 1979; Sharpe, Hermsen and Billings, 2002: 78) and supposedly forced a rethinking of societal norms regarding the division of work and family responsibilities, as well as spotlighting the role of employers in helping employees meet family time demands. Initially, the move to the paid workforce found employed wives and mothers working two shifts (Hochschild, 1989), with women doing a disproportionate amount of household work (Sharpe, Hermsen and Billings, 2002: 79). However, many employers have implemented family-friendly workplace policies designed to help busy workers meet conflicting work and family demands. These workplace policy innovations often involve alternative work arrangements that reconfigure the hours, place and schedule of employment (Sharpe, Hermsen and Billings, 2002: 79). However, for the women in this study with overwhelming, multiple responsibilities, such workplace initiatives fell short. The uncertainty of their child's condition often had a direct impact on their career choices and many of them still had to 'do it all'.

Work choices and their outcomes were heavily influenced by this context. Wendy shared that her daughter's illness had impacted her career choices and decisions. For instance, career investments routinely undertaken by colleagues became precariously anticipated by her:

Wendy: I suppose I've been most affected from last December, when I was going to a conference and Samantha collapsed for a

week and was really sick. And I had to decide whether to go to the conference or stay at home, and whether or not she'd be able to join me ... at the second conference. [Samantha] ended up spending a week with my daughter ... and then did join me ...
Researcher: You must have felt really uncomfortable making that decision.
Wendy: Oh, it was really, really hard. Yes ... It had all been set up for her to stay with a friend, go to school, all that sort of thing. It was *all* handled. And then the night before, she just went pfft. So, yes, it was really difficult. (Wendy, Interview 1: 5)

Charlene also pointed to the choices she had made restricting her career. Charlene, like Wendy, was well-qualified and capable. Unfortunately, for her, the flexibility she needed to care for her paraplegic son limited the work possibilities. The result? She was not financially well set up for the future:

> **Researcher:** Do you feel that this limited your career in any way, and your life opportunities?
> **Charlene:** Yes, extremely. I have no pension. I have *nothing* for myself.
> **Researcher:** It's probably a hard question, but if Jamie hadn't been paraplegic, where would you have been today career-wise?
> **Charlene:** I would have hoped that the last –, that I would be some place in a company where I would be middle management to upper management, and be established in that company.
> **Researcher:** You have an MBA?
> **Charlene:** Yes. (Charlene, Interview 1: 8)

Hancock (2002: 122) confirms that casual employment carries fewer rights, benefits and entitlements, although some casual workers who are able to prove continuity of work can access a patchwork of entitlements. Unfortunately, Charlene's story revealed that she had been unable to do this. She represented the more likely outcome of casual employees at the bottom end of the occupational spectrum, vulnerable to low pay and multiple forms of employment insecurity; insecurities that include tenure, income, work hours and representation (Hancock, 2002: 122; Campbell, 2000). And casual employment is spreading from those groups where it has been traditional (i.e. full-time students and women) to prime working age males as the availability of full-time jobs diminishes. Charlene and Oitk both opted for part-time work deliberately to give them the flexibility they needed. Kurz (2000: 444) confirms that many mothers work (multiple) part-time jobs because it gives them the flexibility in work hours they seek, including being at home when the children return from school (Kurz, 2000: 444).

I was very concerned about these choices and the likely life, career and financial limitations that could arise as a result, especially when combined with the additional responsibilities that these women endured. I constructed Vignette 8 to explore how these women positioned their careers and work choices alongside their caring responsibilities:

> **Vignette 8: Career, promotions, opportunities**
> You have just received an email asking for qualified people to apply for a job. This job will suit your qualifications and experience perfectly, but will also provide additional challenges that you feel ready and confident to take on. This is your dream job. It will also be paying you almost double your current salary.
>
> Then you notice that a significant amount of travel will be required. You will be required to travel interstate and overseas one week in every 4–6 weeks. This will be a regular requirement of the role. You will also have to work late regularly.
>
> Will you apply? Why or why not? What factors did you consider when making your decision? How do you feel about your choice? (Vignette 8, see Appendix)

Sally reported that she would not have applied for this job:

> **Researcher:** Would you apply? Why or why not?
> **Sally:** No probably not. While these opportunities don't happen often I feel that they will come again. Now is not the right time. I might if I had good support at home and others that could take on those responsibilities. It may be something that, financially, we need to do as a family, to take up the opportunity.
> **Researcher:** How do you feel about your choice? ...
> **Sally:** Disappointed – and philosophical. Shit happens and life sucks sometimes. (Sally, Interview 2: 4)

Sally's pithy and disappointed response highlighted a number of issues. First, her responsibilities at home precluded her from applying.

Women do adjust their work obligations through reduced job status and decisions to take less demanding positions (Gjerdingen et al, 2000: 13). They may also choose to cut back on job commitments or take periods of leave if needed. However, such decisions contribute to women remaining underrepresented in administrative and managerial positions, and overrepresented in clerical and service occupations (Gjerdingen et al, 2000: 13). The amount of travel and the long hours indicated in the fictional job – Sally's dream job – she felt, would not allow her to do all that she needed to do for her family. Sally also indicated that such an opportunity may present itself in the future; that 'now was not the right time'. However, given that Sally's daughter was 16 years old at the time of interview, I wondered when (and if?) the right time might ever emerge? Finally, and of great interest, Sally stated she did not currently have adequate support at home to enable her to do this job. In order for her to return to work full-time, Sally had told me that she had negotiated with her family what her return to work would mean for them; chores were shared out and everyone in her family learned that she wasn't going to be as available to them as she had been previously.

However, despite these negotiations, she obviously still believed that any further work-related infringements on her time and energy were not possible. And her poignant response? 'Shit happens and life sucks sometimes'. While we see her disappointment handled so eloquently, I wondered why she could not have returned to her family and renegotiated their respective roles, especially the division of home responsibilities between her and her partner. As a full-time working woman, with a disability and limitations myself, I lamented that Sally felt unable to elicit the support she needed from her family. I also wondered if some of the responsibility for the lack of support might reside with Sally herself. While acknowledging the enormous socialised pressure on Sally to put her family first and put her needs last, Sally had impressed me as an assertive, strident and confident woman. I hope that her reflections on this in the future might have prompted new ways of thinking – for her and her family – enabling her to respond to future career opportunities if they arose in a more positive fashion. Wendy indicated a similar philosophical response when she chose not to apply for promotion when the opportunity arose:

> **Researcher:** What effect has Samantha's illness had on your work-life, say, over the last three years? [slight pause] I'm thinking about choices, work choices, work undertaken, those sorts of things?

Wendy: Probably in the last two years, not a great deal. You know, there's been the doctors' appointments and because of the flexibility of my hours, I've been able to work from home, juggle work over a 24-hour period and a seven-day period. In that sense, I'm not chained to the 'forty hours in the public service' like I was, for example. So in that sense, I'm in an occupation that has enormous flexibility ... I suppose in the last year, partly because work was so busy and partly also I had a lot on my plate, I didn't apply for promotion ... It actually went past me before I even knew. And I can't say that was just family. Certainly this time, I'm not applying for promotion: one, because I think it would be better to do it next year and, two, I've had far too much on my plate because of my daughter being sick. (Wendy, Interview 1: 4–5)

Wendy pointed to her opportunity to apply for promotion having gone 'past' her. Her work choices (or creeping nonchoices) had affected her career over the short and long-term. Without applying for promotion, Wendy was never going to progress. However, it was easy to see why she couldn't summon the physical and emotional energy to put together an application. As we have seen throughout this book, just keeping going was, sometimes, all these women could do.

8
Survival, Compassion and Action

Work Blurs with Home

A performance difficulty
Talk to them
Empathy: What might be causing certain things?
Personal lives at work; work blurs with home.

At some point, a clear discussion
It's becoming performance-related
You've done great work; you're capable of great work
You need help.

Thank you for sharing
Do you need to take some time?
Great empathy
An employer can be supportive.

But still an obligation as a manager
Meet them half way
Consideration, but they own responsibility
Work blurs with home.

(Dolly, Interview 2: 20–21)

Back to the beginning

To conclude this volume, I return to the original research question, exploring briefly the substantive and methodological questions that I sought to answer, as well as reflecting on what has been learned and how it has paved the way for future knowledge in this area. The next section illustrates the positive outcomes reported in this research journey. I then discuss the need to return to compassion, in workplaces and communities, before offering some concluding comments regarding the actionable knowledge achieved to date, and sought for the future.

You will recall that this research journey commenced to answer the following question:

> What is life like for a full-time worker who also cares for a child with a chronic illness?

In responding to this question, I hope to have opened the door to understanding. I tried to do this in a way that was at once rigorous and yet artistic. I tried to make it interesting, informative and artful; an enticement to readers. We have learned that these women felt disconnected from others and had to do it all; we saw their grief and loss; the cruelty and thoughtlessness of others; the lack of support, and their resultant career choices and limitations. However, I was also concerned substantively with: (1) how well the research methods provided the data sought; and (2) whether the data gathered answered the research question. As I reflect on what has been shared here, I believe that the methods employed worked well. I delved into the 'mess' of these women's lives in an effort to improve the human condition. I fed back the findings to respondents along the way, and demonstrated what Fricke (2004) eloquently described as the 'field talking back'. Respondents responded to their own reflections; they responded to the vignettes I created; and they responded to my interpretations. The data outcomes were rich and varied, telling and showing how life was for the women who participated in this study, while also providing the impetus for future social change. I hope that the combination of texts has proven as evocative and rewarding to read as it was to write, and write about.

I also wanted to reflect, methodologically, about the research process: (1) how well the use of retrospective and prospective interviewing worked; (2) how useful the fictional vignettes were; and (3) whether the Culminating Group Experience (CGE) achieved its aims. From my perspective, the offerings in this volume depict the successful use of retrospective and prospective interviewing. The different orientations helped me learn what had happened, and what could change and be improved for the future. The vignettes allowed me to confirm respondent responses to certain situations that I had learned about in the Stage 1 interviews. I knew how I felt about what had been described to me, but I was able, by reflecting similar situations back to those similarly placed, to learn if my assumptions and responses were appropriate and aligned with theirs. Finally, the CGE also achieved most of its aims, which were to (1) generate discussion; (2) learn more about the accuracy or otherwise of my interpretations; (3) find out about respondents' experiences of participating in this research; and (4) provide opportunities for respondents to network. Certainly, lively discussion was generated which enabled me to learn if my interpretations were reasonably accurate or not, and how they might be further developed. While few respondents were able to attend, limiting the networking opportunities I had hoped for, I was able to learn about their experience as a participant in this research by asking what they thought. Evalyn shared this:

> **Researcher:** Is there anything else that this has brought up that you'd like to talk about or anything that ... you wanted to share?
> **Evalyn:** Yes. I still remember getting very teary and upset in the first interview, and it's something that obviously I hadn't –, I thought I'd resolved a lot of things, but obviously there are still things that cut deep to the bone. But I'm glad, I'm really glad to have participated in this and I really looked forward to this, Margaret. I've really enjoyed talking about things and Kevin. It gives me a chance to reflect and gives me a chance of thinking about –, you're so busy with day-to-day life and then you realise that sometimes you do feel guilty. I got a letter from Kevin's speech pathologist yesterday saying, 'Despite numerous times of trying to contact you ...' [laughter]. But, you know, I don't think it's unreasonable for me to want to work.
> **Researcher:** Yes, that's right.
> **Evalyn:** You know ... if I had decided to devote my whole life – just 24/7 to my children – then that's doing a disservice to *me*. Kevin is a big part of my life, but he's not my *whole* life and I think you have to see that ... it's all about balance. It's not unreasonable to want to work and to contribute in other ways. (Evalyn, Interview 2: 19–20)

I was thrilled to hear her reflections, and tremendously grateful to Evalyn for sharing her views. Regarding the vignettes, Evalyn confirmed their representational accuracy:

> **Evalyn:** I thought they were very realistic. I thought these things will certainly happen and are certainly issues for people who have

disability in their family, and I could very easily picture myself in any of these vignettes. (Evalyn, Interview 2: 9)

Finally, with regard to the CGE, both respondents who attended reported that they felt better knowing that they were not alone in their circumstances. When Wendy suggested that 'some people have it much worse' (Wendy, CGE: 1), Evalyn agreed:

Evalyn: Yes. And it makes you realise that you're not alone, which is really important. Because I guess, among your family and friends, you are a minority. And so you don't get to see and hear of other people who have the same kind of experiences. So it's really wonderful to get that. (Evalyn, CGE: 1; Vickers, 2005e: 211)

The project also resulted in learning and behaviour change for these women. Evalyn demonstrated her learning about mothers taking on the majority of the work, of 'doing it all'. She also reported being surprised that she was one of the few respondents in a supportive partner relationship. Concurrently, she recognised, for the first time, that her partner had been 'supplementing' her efforts, rather than sharing them equally:

Evalyn: Yes. I totally agree with your finding, at the end, that mothers do tend to have the primary caregiving role and the father is seen as a supplement, almost like a supplementary kind of care-giver. And I was really surprised at how many negative cases you found where the father was almost detrimental to the caregiving process, and wasn't really supportive or anything. I guess I was very lucky in that respect, because my husband has been very supportive and caring. And I know a family where it *has* split them up. So I guess I'm lucky in that respect. But I was surprised that it was almost like a minority. (Evalyn, CGE: 2; Vickers, 2005e: 212)

Evalyn had learned from these dialogues new insights into her partner relationship. She also expressed the positive and practical outcome of finding she was not alone in her experiences – an awaken-ing in itself. While this new knowledge may or may not have resulted in behavioural changes for Evalyn – *actionable* knowledge in the prag-matic, physical sense – it was still learning that resulted in the very real outcome of making her feel more content, comfortable and comforted. While acknowledging a new perspective on her partner relationship, she also felt more appreciative of her partner's contributions and support, in light of her learning of others' experiences. Such an outcome was very valuable. Evalyn's concluding commentary included her ambivalent response to my presentation of the emergent themes and stories from other women:

> **Evalyn:** I felt when we were actually reading, telling us about your experience in your studies, it was kind of really sad. I felt really sad. And I, you know, I felt like crying a couple of times at how sad some of these stories were. But right now, talking here right now, I feel quite positive. You know, it's how you deal with the situation. (Evalyn, CGE: 6–7; Vickers, 2005e: 212)

The knowledge-generating dialogue that was created in the CGE resulted in Evalyn, ultimately, feeling very positive. For her, the improvement and innovation in her life lay with acknowledging the plight of others, talking about and sharing her own experiences and challenges, and knowing that she was dealing effectively and positively with what life had handed her. The creation of positive feelings, including increased self-efficacy, was a worthy actionable knowledge outcome indeed.

As noted earlier, not all the experiences reported by respondents were negative. Some were very positive indeed and it is important that such expressions of positive support, happiness, pride and joy be acknowledged. Below are stories of survival that should not be forgotten:

- Surviving at work;
- Surviving with people;
- Surviving by living; and
- The surviving self.

The stories portrayed these women's survival, enhanced by their own actions and choices, and by the friendship, caring and generosity of those around them, at work and elsewhere. They deserve attention, especially when considering the path ahead.

Surviving at work

In terms of survival, the workplace was one area where these women demonstrated their consummate ability to find their way through difficult circumstances. Surviving at work meant making choices that were enabling and self-supporting. You will recall (see Chapter 3) that all respondents were the first point of call for any emergency with their child or if assistance was required by schools or carers. Sandra, Wendy, Evalyn, Sally, Dolly and Oitk all reported that they were the ones first contacted by their child's school if there was a problem. Dolly, Oitk, Evalyn and Cate also reported doing lengthy stints staying with their children at hospital when it was required. As a result of these responsibilities, almost without exception, respondents reported gravitating towards work and career choices that enabled them to maintain significant amounts of flexibility in *doing* their work. This might have included the hours they worked, where they worked, or the type of work they chose.

For instance, Dolly was able to retain the much required flexibility she needed by working in a human resources (HR) consulting business – her own. Similarly, Sandra was the managing director of her own personnel placement agency; Evalyn and Polly worked in the public sector, choices that meant significant drops in salary, but much greater flexibility in terms of flexi-time and the ability to work at home if the need arose; and Wendy was able to work at home when she needed to, confirming her orientation to a work environment that allowed her to cope with the demands brought by her daughter's chronic illness. Charlene chose part-time work to enable the flexibility she needed to maintain her caring responsibilities while still providing income for her family. These women chose flexible work environments, which allowed them to take control of their lives – and survive. Cate confirmed that her workplace survival was enhanced by her choice of working in the disability services sector:

> **Researcher:** And as far as William's impact on your work life, is there a positive or negative impact? Has it affected where you wanted to be and what you wanted to do?
> **Cate:** Yes, it has. Not in a bad way. This place is pretty open about if I had to take time off, and to work with him. It's been really good because I learned a lot about funding services and stuff like that, because there's the fact that I work here. But if I didn't work here, I don't know that I would have that kind of help. It's been really helpful ... When he was first born, they actually let me bring him here for about six months. They let me have him here for a few hours each day, which was really cool. If they weren't so receptive, I'd probably have to address it, but I can't imagine that they'd ever

say to me, 'You can't do this because of the needs of your son', because that's who we serve. (Cate, Interview 1: 5)

Orientations to flexible working arrangements were hardly surprising. However, there are two important points to consider. First, orienting to flexible work arrangements may well have deleterious effects on careers, lives and finances, especially in the long-term. Second, just because flexibility in work options was achieved, life did not necessarily become 'easy' – just possible.

Surviving with people

A notable area that aided these women's survival was the kindness and thoughtfulness of others. Not everyone they came into contact with was thoughtless and cruel; some were very helpful and kind. Respondents portrayed people in their lives who really helped 'keep them sane' and had supported them – pragmatically, physically, emotionally or financially. Sally referred, for example, to her friend's pragmatic advice, which Sally often sought, regarding her daughter's well-being; Sandra and Dolly spoke highly of friends and colleagues who supported them; Charlene was touched by the kindness of a stranger:

> **Researcher:** Have you ever felt different because of Jamie?
> **Charlene:** ... There were times. One time at Christmas, I had no money. We were in this toy store looking for some toys, and I was looking at the 99-cent ones. And the lady came up and she said, 'I would like to buy your son some Christmas presents. My grandson just died, and I need to buy some Christmas presents'. And she bought him toys.
> **Researcher:** That's a lovely story ...
> **Charlene:** It was very tempting to say, 'No'. [Weeping] Because I couldn't afford the toys myself, and I couldn't buy them for my daughter. But I said, 'Yes', not because my son needed the toys, but because *she* needed to buy them. (Charlene, Interview 1: 7)

Sally also recalled the loving gift from a friend, that brought tears to her eyes – and mine:

> **Sally:** But friends were –, everybody rallied around and supported us. One girlfriend from work, she came, and she'd lost her daughter

a few years earlier; she was hit by a car. She came with this present, a little thing. She said, 'It's not something new', and it was actually her daughter's bracelet, because her daughter was born with all her internal organs on the outside. So she's endured that, survived that, and then got hit by a car many years later. She said, 'It brought Elizabeth good luck; I want you to have it for Nadine'. And I just cried again. I still actually have that. I still have that. (Sally, Interview 1: 14)

Surviving by living

While many respondents indicated fairly serious changes to their lives, either directly or indirectly, as a result of their child's disability, they were also able to appreciate and enjoy the serendipitous and pleasing outcomes that manifested in their lives. For example, while Cate talked about how her child's disability prevented the family from going out to eat or to the movies, she was able to draw on the positive, and was pleased about learning to be such a good cook:

Cate: Well, family outings is one thing, because of the fact that he's unpredictable. I mean, I tried to get him socialised as far as going out to eat and stuff like that, but it's just too hard. We don't even go out any more. Consequently, I got to be a good cook. *That's* cool. (Cate, Interview 1: 23)

Respondents also reported many different ways of dealing with their overwhelming circumstances. I was struck by the fact that, even in the face of all their challenges, they all pressed on, remained philosophical about their lot, and indicated a refusal to dwell on the negative side of things. Some were also creative: Sally liked 'scrapbooking'; Cate reported numerous artistic activities that she clearly enjoyed:

Cate: Well, there's a lot of things that I like to do that don't have to do with this job. Like my art, and I play drums in a band and stuff like that. I know it sounds crazy, but I do. And it's been really fun. I've played drums for about 14 years now. We have this wild band. Colin and I – that's my husband – that's kind of a bonding thing that we do. It's really important to us.
Researcher: You and your husband bonding?
Cate: Yes, totally. He plays guitar and writes the songs, and I can write some songs too, but mostly I just play drums. And the kids like

it too, because William, he wants to sit and play drums, and we do that like a rock-and-roll family. (Cate, Interview 1: 5–6)

The surviving self

Others reported positive outlets that were initiated by themselves, for themselves. For example, Dolly reported that she had recently lost 20 kilograms in weight, a tremendous achievement. She was walking every morning and feeling great about it all. She hastened to add that this weight had crept on over years of rushing meals and not finding time to exercise and look after herself. While Sandra reported having gained weight and not taken enough time for herself, smoking and drinking (although not a great deal), and nibbling on peanuts in the evenings, especially when under stress (Sandra, Interview 1: 7), she also balanced this with seeing a 'life coach' who helped her with energy channeling and other alternative therapies to reduce the stress and tension in her life. Sandra also reported getting regular massages to reduce tension. Wendy reported similarly proactive, positive behaviours:

> **Researcher:** What sort of things do you do to cope? You mentioned going along to EAP [Employee Assistance Program] at [Wendy's workplace]. What do you do – positive and negative?
> **Wendy:** I definitely eat too much – that's one. Watch television. Use the research, find out stuff. Incredibly, really find out stuff. I go through phases of that … What else? I'm too tired to read. I garden; I walk; I try to make time to go out and do something once a weekend, which is really nice.
> **Researcher:** So you're obviously conscious of looking after yourself.
> **Wendy:** Oh yes. Yes. And do a little bit of retail therapy, but not much [laughter]. (Wendy, Interview 1: 18–19)

Sally reported that, for her, successful coping was enhanced by the simple act of getting a good night's sleep. I asked her:

> **Researcher:** In terms of looking after yourself, what do you do to keep your head together and to keep going? …
> **Sally:** At the moment, I don't have time to do anything. I like scrap-booking; that's just something new I've discovered in the last couple of years. Love that … If I don't get time, well I just don't get to it. At the moment, university work is the priority because there are dead-lines to meet and that kind of stuff. I make sure I go to bed; I tend

to get into bed at a reasonable hour, because if I get an alright night's sleep, I can cope with anything, and have always pretty much been like that. I think it's even more important now with the workload, the study load, the family stuff, that I make sure that happens. (Sally, Interview 1: 26)

The respondents demonstrated, repeatedly, their own selves as a source and means of survival. I move now to consider the future. What might be done in response to what has been learned?

Towards compassion

What Do I Say?

I'd give this lady a big hug
That's the first thing I'd do
I know how this is; I know how this would be.

What do I say?
I'd just say, 'You have to hang in there'
She's been through it before; she can do it again.

What's the biggest fear?
That the child is going to die
That's the biggest fear.

Just be there for this person, let her talk
Let her know you're thinking about her
That's what you do.

(Evalyn, Interview 2: 17)

One way forward is through the compassion of others. Extending the work of Dutton et al (2002), where the notion of the compassionate workplace is introduced, I believe individuals at all levels in organisations and communities should be encouraged to develop a *Context for Meaning*, where an environment is facilitated so that people can freely express and discuss the way they feel, what they are feeling, and seek the understanding and support they may require. In addition to meaning, comes the development of a *Context of Action*. Again, individuals at all levels in the organisation and community should be encouraged to acknowledge the suffering and difficulties of others, and to help them seek the assistance they require to move forward proactively and positively. This all begins with ending the silence on troubled lives, such as the lives of these women. Acknowledging anguish and enabling survival are themes reflected throughout this book. These women frequently demonstrated their refusal to be silenced, their propensity to accept the challenges that faced them, pragmatically and without drama, and to challenge aspects of their lives they did not consider satisfactory and to try to change them. They sought a life where their challenges, fear and pain should not be silenced. A family, workplace and a community that acknowledges grief and facilitates understanding and support would be a positive start – and is long overdue.

Towards actionable knowledge

Another positive step towards the future – towards actionable knowledge – and one of the major purposes of this work, is to support what is defined as 'participatory competence'; that is, the ability to be heard by those in power (Kieffer, 1984; Gibson, 1995: 1208). Parents of children with long-term health conditions need to be supported by those who can help; those in power, including those in the community and their places of work. They also need to be heard by families, friends, and professional service providers. More evidence is required about current levels of unmet needs in children and their families in Australia (Martin and Nisa, 1996). It is especially vital to consider the needs of working parents – especially working mothers – for social support, both at home and at work, both formal and informal. Increasing participatory competence (Kieffer, 1984; Gibson, 1995: 1208) is most likely to be achieved via attention to intrapersonal factors, such as the values, beliefs, determination and the experience of mothers in these roles (Gibson, 1995: 1209). Improved social support is very valuable in encouraging individual empowerment (Gibson, 1995: 1209).

Actionable knowledge at the local level (see Chapter 2) has been demonstrated. Dolly was losing weight; Sandra had realised her role in letting her partner distance himself emotionally from her family's needs; Wendy was 'handing things back', getting her partner involved in her daughter's medication procurement; Polly had moved to a public sector position, a deliberate choice taking her away from high power and time-consuming jobs of her fast-track past; Oitk had resigned from a job she found stressful to permit her studies to continue; and Evalyn recognised that, while supportive, her partner had been supplementing her efforts rather than equalling them. These women had taken matters into their own hands; they were surviving as a result of their own skills, reflections and endeavours. The dialogues we had prompted their reflection and learning, as well as the development of 'local theory' as an important foundation for action (Palshaugen, 2004b: 184). However, and importantly, the respondents also demonstrated changes in knowledge of their own situations, enabling them to create action plans that resulted in pragmatic, meaningful action to improve their lives.

Another of the objectives of this project (described in Chapter 2) was to find out if it was necessary and feasible to carry out a larger one. This was confirmed with this research project bringing a previously underresearched area into the spotlight. The local knowledge and researcher interpretations have been utilised to improve the human condition. On a larger scale, the exploratory work undertaken in the study reported here also served to support a successful application for an Australian Research Council Linkage Grant to fund a national study into the support needs of parents of children with chronic illness. This is now underway. Hence, knowledge from this exploratory study was a catalyst for the specifics of this practical problem being addressed on a wider scale. From local theory comes local actionable knowledge applied in a very pragmatic way, and on a much larger scale. In this case, the larger research project will uncover more detailed information, quantitative and qualitative, about the support needs of full-time workers caring for a child with chronic illness, across Australia. Greenwood (2002) confirms that action research need not just include qualitative studies. Specifically, the outcomes of this larger study will include: enhanced understanding of the support needs of full-time workers who care for a child with chronic illness; qualitative and quantitative data to inform policy makers, healthcare providers, employers, educators, and healthcare professionals to provide more proactive, responsive and responsible social support and information services; and, a validated, sensitive survey questionnaire that will provide empirical data about the support needs of people who work full-time and care for a child with chronic illness. Hence, the impetus and action for social change continues.

I share Gustavsen's (2004: 163) sentiments on the worthwhile nature of longer-term projects, especially in terms of their capacity to expand into different discourses and lines of discovery. The likelihood of social change can be enhanced with some preparedness of action researchers to deliberately include the gathering of 'scientific' and 'objective' data – data that is routinely insisted upon by decision makers (and might often be outside the action research arena) – as part of *their means to effect change.* As Greenwood (2002: 131) insists, conducting good research means developing habits of counterintuitive thinking, linking findings and processes located in other cases, and attempting to subject our interpretations to outside critique. Taking this project forward in a more positivist direction is, for me, taking up such a challenge.

I leave you by inviting you to read the Epilogue to this book. This was written as an alternative to the fictional diary entry shared in the Introduction. I still had the respondents in mind when I wrote it. I asked myself, as I wrote, how could their day be easier? What might they need to change, in themselves and in others? How might a small change in one part of their lives flow in and around the rest of their lives with a 'ripple effect' of betterment? Whatever can be done to improve the lives of these women must be done. I had in mind that imagining a brighter future, through informed fiction development, might serve to assist the journey forward to a better means of survival, through compassion and action.

Epilogue: Creating a New Story?

Dear Diary

The alarm punches me awake. While as reluctant as ever to move out from under the covers, this morning I feel quite good. David has stopped having seizures during the night. A simple change in his medication has changed all our lives. More sleep means that I can handle just about any-thing! I say good morning to David, and to Susan, his new carer, who is preparing breakfast for us both, and head for the shower.

Since joining the support group being run for working carers in our local community, I learned, from one of the other mothers, that there is a new anti-seizure medication out now that has worked wonders controlling her son's multiple seizures. After I spoke with the neurologist, we gave it a go. And now, more often than not, David sleeps through the night. That means I get a good night's sleep too. And because he sleeps better, he is less susceptible to every cold and flu going around. Such a small change, but what a big effect.

I hear Susan fussing quietly in the kitchen with David, playing with him and getting his breakfast. She is just fantastic. I learned about her via a website for working carers. She is a uni student studying nursing and it suits her to earn some money this way early in the mornings. The support group and the website are a great source of information. The website actually has a list of potential carers available that they claim to be professional, reliable and available. And there is a list to choose from; if I am not especially happy with one, I have others to choose from. They range in the services available too, from full-time, live-in, nanny services, to early mornings, afternoons, evenings and weekends. And Susan has just been great. She comes to get David ready for school four mornings a week, 6–8 am. This means that, not only can I sleep a little later, I can still get to work a bit earlier and start my day more reliably. That is quite a relief. Another carer, Jenny, is available to pick David up from school at 3.30 pm and I take over in the evening, when I get home at around 6 pm. By the time I get home, David is bathed and fed, dinner is prepared for me, and I get some playtime with my son before he goes off to bed. I can then, all being well, have some 'me-time' as I eat dinner, do some reading or watch a DVD or TV, before getting to bed at a reasonable hour, sleeping through the night and being able to get up for the next day. How things have changed!

My mother and I have found a new place in our relationship probably aided by my not always having to ask her to drop everything, including her favoured bingo and bridge club get-togethers, to look after David when I can't find anyone else at short notice. When the now rare occasions arise that I do ask, she is far more receptive. She even congratulated me the other day, noting how organised and relaxed I seemed to be these days. Finally, another unanticipated positive: she now wants to come and see David and I for social visits. Our relationship has certainly changed for the better. We now find time to chat about the usual stuff; family, politics, David, her, me, TV celebrities, and what's happening in our favourite soap opera (that I now have time to watch!)

And work has improved too. I made a conscious choice to rearrange my work schedule. I now start a little earlier, around 7.30 am, and still finish around 5.30 pm, for four days per week. I have, deliberately, cut back to four days per week (still full-time, but four longer days), so that I might have a mid-week 'break'. I stay at home on Wednesday, catching up on emails and paperwork, as required, but being sure to at least leave the afternoon totally free – for me. I walk regularly (and also do this on weekends as well) and find that I am losing weight. Encouraged by this, I have cut back on the evening chocolate solace (now only one night per week), which is also helping. The weight loss and the regular exercise, along with feeling more rested and organised, has found in me a renewed interest in shopping for clothes. It is always pleasing to be able to slide into that smaller dress size! Interestingly, all these changes have also found me performing better at work. My sales figures are higher than they have been for ages, and colleagues and clients find me far more reliable (and productive, when I am present). Consequently, I have more money to spend on myself, on David, and on the carers that I need. Work is more satisfying than it has been for a long-time and has shifted away from being just drudgery and effort.

Things with my ex-husband, Jack, have also improved. Several months ago, when I was ready to explode or fall apart (I wasn't sure which, but *thought it would be ugly, either way), I rang him one evening in tears. I just had to talk to him and get some more help from him. 'After all', I said, 'David is your son too!' While Jack can be a bit insensitive and thoughtless in some ways, I know that he loves and cares for David very much. Since we separated, we have always been able to put David's needs ahead of our other issues. Thankfully, Jack stepped up. He came around to see me and, over a glass of wine, we discussed how he could become more involved with David's life and how this might help take some of the load off me. He now takes David every second weekend, for most school holidays, and also picks him up from school on Wednesday afternoon (my day off), dropping him back to me Wednesday evening, bathed, fed and ready for bed. Jack also keeps sets of sheets, pyjamas, and clothes for David at his house and handles all the washing and maintenance required when he is there. No more bags of washing returned for me to do. He also keeps back up medication there, so there is less for me to organise. So, as Jack is living quite close now, this is working out really well. David loves spending more time with Jack – and vice versa. Jack has always been great with David. And, well, I am not exactly unhappy about it either – my time with David is much more fun and far more relaxed these days.*

I have to say that, while problems do arise still – David still does have the occasional seizure, even during the night, and he still gets the routine childhood illnesses that make everyone in the household miserable – I am now not desperate when it happens. I have a number of pleasant, professional and reliable carers I can call upon that David is happy being around and that I am comfortable having in our home. I now find, my mother is so much closer to me emotionally, and so is Jack. I don't feel so alone now and find time to catch up with friends that I haven't seen for years. I don't think Jack and I will ever get back together – too much has happened – but at least I know I can rely on him, more and more, for pragmatic and emotional support where caring for David is concerned. The more time he spends with David – doing everything that needs to be done for him – the more competent and confident he becomes. And the more relaxed I am with all of it. I now find time to go to the community support group and to exchange emails with other parents similarly placed because of that website I found. I have also become rather friendly with one of the other fathers in this group – a single man caring for a child with autism. Who knows where that might lead?

Finally, I have found that the relationship with the school David attends has improved. This, of course, is because I have time to attend events, like swimming days, and school concerts. I can, if necessary, change my Wednesday 'off day' for special occasions. It is a hassle – but it is possible. I am no longer this distant, shadowy figure who purports to be David's caring mother. I am a far more active participant because I have more time and more energy. Granted, life is rather structured, but I have far more support, and more time, money and energy to get on with my life. Apart from doing well at work, another welcome source of additional financial support comes from the government: thanks to the website I found, I now know what financial support is available to me, and am making use of this to assist with things like childcare and medication. I just never had the time, the knowledge or the energy to check these things out before. This will save me quite a bit of money over the long-term.

As I dress for work, sliding into my new suit and feeling energised and excited about my early morning sales presentation, I reflect on how much things have changed. Much of it has been of my making and I am proud of that. However, I also realise that I could not be doing what I am doing without the help of those around me. I just could not. I kiss David goodbye and, as I wipe the inevitable smear of jam off my cheek and smile, I thank Susan again for her help and head off, ready for the day ahead.

Bring it on!

Appendix: Fictional Vignettes

Vignette 1: Support and other assistance

You are a senior manager in a large finance company. This organisation has many 'family-friendly' policies, but is also currently involved in a large-scale restructure and retrenchment programme. You have an employee working for you who has had a lot of leave since she has worked there. In fact, it is something that you have been meaning to speak to her about. You need to explain to her that her job is in jeopardy because of the perception around the place that she is 'not pulling her weight'. Other than that, you have found her a great asset to the place. You don't want to lose her.

However, before you speak to her, she approaches you, asking for a confidential meeting. She appears very agitated, is tearful during the discussion. She tells you (for the first time) that she has a teenager who has had difficulties socially and at school for most of the child's life. She has visited every doctor, psychiatrist and psychologist, and yet still it remains unclear what is wrong with this child. The behavioural problems have continued, and even escalated. Then she tells you that her child has just been 'scheduled' (admitted without consent) to the local psychiatric hospital, where she is currently under lock and key, and constant observation. This is because her child has just attempted suicide – again. This is the child's third attempt on her own life.

This woman also tells you that her husband has recently left her, and that one of the reasons was that he was 'fed up with dealing with all this' and that he doesn't know what else to do. This woman has no family living locally. She tells you that she doesn't know what to do, how she is going to cope.

As her manager, what do you say to her – and why? How do you feel about doing/saying this? What else are you thinking/feeling?

Vignette 2: Cruelty, thoughtlessness, managerialism

You are at work, in a meeting with one of your senior managers. You receive a phone call, telling you that your child has been sent home from school/ childcare, with a very high temperature. You have previously told this manager of the health problems your child experiences, as you have had to leave work in a hurry previously. You tell your manager what has happened, anticipating a supportive comment and an invitation to leave immediately to see your child. Instead, he proceeds to give you a lengthy lecture about the importance of leaving your 'home' problems at home. He then asks you how often is 'this sort of thing' likely to keep happening?

What do you say? How would that influence your feelings about working there in the future? For example, would you (could you) leave? Would you complain about his behaviour to anyone at work?

Vignette 3: Emotions in the workplace

You are at work and notice that one of your junior female colleagues is very distracted and agitated. You ask her if she is all right. Does she need some help? She immediately starts to cry.

She confesses to you that she has a child with an intellectual disability and, also, a serious childhood cancer. The child has just been rushed to hospital with a high fever and is unconscious. Your colleague is frantic. She asks her manager if she can leave work to go to the hospital, to have this time off without pay (she had already used up all her sick leave and annual leave).

Her manager, who already knew of her child's condition, reluctantly said she could go. However, the manager also commented that if she left work – again – on such short notice, she may as well not bother coming back. Her manager complained that he was sick of her rushing off like this all the time, adding that if she were 'able to think rationally about all this' she would see that maybe it would be best for all concerned if the child didn't regain consciousness.

What would you say to your friend? What else would you do (if anything)? How does this make *you* feel?

Vignette 4: Relationships

Part I

You are a single mum. You have been working at your current workplace for some time. You enjoy your work and are coping as best you can with caring for your child on your own. You have only told one person – in confidence – about your child's disability at your work.

Recently, you have developed a particular friendship with one of your single male colleagues. You like him a lot. The two of you have started to regularly 'do lunch'. You have found that he was married for about three years, but has recently divorced. He has no children from that marriage. He suggests a meal out together and you accept immediately then retreat into a personal panic, as you wonder who will babysit your child. You also wonder when, and how, you are going to tell him about your child.

What do you do?

Part II

You ask your very understanding mother to babysit for you – again – on this special occasion. However, she warns that she is 73 and can't be expected to care for your child all week after school while you are working *and* on the weekends while you go off partying.

You go to dinner and have a great time. You decide that you need to tell him about your child but are nervous about his reaction.

What do you do?

Part III

Well, it seems that you don't need to tell him, because your 'friend' at work – who you confided in about your sick child – has already done so. She has been noticing you and 'Mr Right' lunching together regularly, fancied 'Mr Right' herself, and decided to let him in on your 'secret' before you had a chance to. You know this, because Mr Right mentioned it to another person at the office, who then came and asked you if it was 'true what they had heard about your *poor little darling?'* and *'How awful!'*

Not only has Mr Right not called or asked you to lunch since you had dinner (this is now two weeks later), you are feeling like an outcast. Everyone is whispering about you, feeling sorry for you, and now talking about your child as if he is some kind of a 'freak'. As you are leaving the office one evening, Mr Right is leaving at the same time. You ask if he enjoyed your evening out. He is very uncomfortable and says that he has to go. You see Mr Right and your 'friend' lunching together the next day.

How do you feel? What would you do (if anything)?

Vignette 5: Feeling different, alone

Part I

A new lady has just started at your office. She seems very nice. The two of you are working together on some projects and start to chat over coffee. She confides in you that she has a child with a learning disability. He is 12 years old. She left her last workplace because she was not given any consideration by her manager, especially if she asked for time off at short notice.

How do you feel? What do you say to her? What advice would you give to her, thinking carefully about all of your workplaces, past and present?

Part II

At your work there is a big annual, staff barbeque coming up. All the families and children are invited. Everyone is going to be there, even senior management. You are coming up for promotion very soon, and have been encouraged strongly by senior staff and publicly praised for your recent achievements.

Does senior management know about your child? Will you take your child to the barbeque? Will you talk with your new friend about it, or decide on your own?

Vignette 6: Financial assistance

You have recently become friends with a woman you work with, who has a child with a chronic condition which has impaired his social development and his learning ability. She tells you that the child is nine years old and is frequently restless, can become very angry, can throw very noisy and very public tantrums, has been known to kick, punch and bite other children when enraged, and has difficulty concentrating. As a result, he has had considerable difficulty learning in the traditional classroom environment.

She tells you that, while he was not *expelled* from the last two schools, on each occasion, it was made clear to her that she had little choice but to find a place for him in another, 'more suitable' learning environment.

She then tells you that she is also, for the same reasons, having difficulty finding anyone who can mind him for any length of time, especially during school holidays. She is also very concerned about the cost of these child-minding services, especially for her child.

What do you suggest? Do you have any suggestions for financial assistance that may help her?

Vignette 7: Disclosure

You have applied for a new job. It is your dream job. You really want this job.

Will you tell them about your child? If yes, who will you tell? At what point will you tell them? Why will you tell them? If not, why not? Might you change your mind in the future? What would change it?

Vignette 8: Career, promotions, opportunities

You have just received an email asking for qualified people to apply for a job. This job will suit your qualifications and experience perfectly, but will also provide additional challenges that you feel ready and confident to take on. This is your dream job. It will also be paying you almost double your current salary.

Then you notice that a significant amount of travel will be required. You will be required to travel interstate and overseas one week in every 4–6 weeks. This will be a regular requirement of the role. You will also have to work late regularly.

Will you apply? Why or why not? What factors did you consider when making your decision? How do you feel about your choice?

Vignette 9: Work flexibility

You are looking for a new job. Your manager is completely unsympathetic to your need to leave right on time every day to be home when your child arrives home from school. She is also completely unsympathetic (she has no children herself) about you having had so much sick leave this year – and has said so many times.

You get a call from a friend you used to work with. She has contacted you because she knows what kind of a performer you are, knows your skills and competencies, and has worked with you in the past. She has a vacancy where she works. This job is very convenient for you: it is very close to home, it is also close to your child's school and the local hospital (which you frequently need to attend with your child), the woman that has rung you knows of the difficulties your child is experiencing and has, in the past, been sympathetic and considerate.

However, this role would not be a step forward in your career. You would earn considerably less money (about 30 per cent less).

What do you do? Why? Did you think about *your child's* financial future when making your choice? How much did this influence your decision? Did you think about *your* financial future when making your choice? How much did this influence your decision?

Vignette 10: Childcare concerns

You have had considerable difficulty finding someone to look after your child during school holidays, and to be there after school when the child arrives home, around 3 pm. However, you find this person in the local paper. She has references and appears knowledgeable (well, a bit) about your child's illness. She is confident with the child, and tells you she has worked as a nurse's aid at a hospital some years ago.

On this particular day, you arrive home from work early. You have just got a promotion and decided to give yourself a reward by taking the rest of the afternoon off. You arrive home and find your child sitting in front of the television in a dirty nappy. This is not just any dirty nappy. It should have been changed *many* hours ago.

Where is your carer? Nowhere to be seen. You notice – for the first time since she started work – a dirty ashtray, full of cigarette butts. You recall asking her if she smoked when you interviewed her for the job, because you didn't want cigarette smoke around your child. She had said no.

About 20 minutes later, the carer arrives home, sees you and is very apologetic. She tells you that she just *had to* get some cigarettes down at the local shop and was only a few moments.

It is Friday, and next week is school holidays.

What do you do? How do you feel? What are you most concerned about – now and in the future?

Vignette 11: Coping

You are just settling in on the couch. It is about 8.30 pm. Your child is asleep at last and, for the first time all day, you feel that your time is your own. You reach for the block of Cadbury and another glass of wine. You are feeling a little bit guilty about this because, after you got the kids a nice healthy dinner, you settled for cheese and crackers, with a few handfuls of cashews for your dinner. You love cashews.

You ponder the fact that the last time you had the courage to get on the scales (weeks ago because it was such a shock), you decided that, this time, you would make a point of eating a healthy diet. You would not be silly about it, but be more careful of what you ate and find some time to do some exercise. You promised yourself to limit the chocolate consumption to one small block, only one night a week, the wine to one glass per day, and to have at least one home prepared meal per day, which included vegetables. You also decided to start walking for 20 minutes every morning. You would start looking after yourself.

This hasn't happened.

Aside from blaming yourself, why else might your new regime not have happened? What can you do about that? What will get you to do that?

Vignette 12: Fear and grief

You are sitting having lunch with a close colleague, a single mum, who has a child with a rare form of cancer. For several years the child has been in remission. You are at the café near your work and having a fun, high-spirited chat, with lots of jokes and fun at your other (less likeable) workmates' expense. You are enjoying your friend's company.

You admire how she copes so well. She seems so strong, so together. She rarely complains about her lot, and if she does, it is always in an upbeat, humorous kind of way. Her child has been through a lot: hospitalisations, drugs, numerous rounds of medical appointments. Your friend has been through it all too and always seems to manage to see the bright side, and find a positive in it all.

You remembered that it is her child's birthday next week. You reach into your bag and pass her a small, brightly-wrapped gift for her to give to the child.

She bursts into tears. Through her tears, you gather that her child's cancer has come back. It is very serious.

What do you do? What do you think is going on here? What do you say? What do you think her biggest fear is? What do you think might help her the most?

Vignette 13: Discrimination (because of your child)

Part I

You decide to apply for a more senior position where you work. You have told a few people about your child's condition at work. You don't even consider that this would be a factor when applying for this great job. You are well-qualified and experienced for this position and are not surprised when you are called for an interview. You go in to the interview feeling very confident.

What does surprise you is this. Towards the end of the interview, one of the interview panel asks you about your family life, specifically if you have any children. He couches this in terms of his own interest in his family and how important balancing home and work is, getting one's priorities straight, with the family coming first, and all that. He asks you specific questions about your children: What are their ages? What do they like to do? You wonder why these questions are being asked. You wonder, in particular, why these questions are being asked now.

You wonder if they know about your child. You are not pleased by these questions – it is none of their business. You are not convinced the interviewer is really the 'family man' that he makes out to be.

What do you say?

Part II

You decide on the spot that you really must tell this interviewer about your family, including (very briefly) the difficulties with your child. You figure that they might have heard about it anyway, so you had better not try to deceive them. However, you then quickly reinforce your other significant and notable qualities and achievements, all achieved with your family responsibilities. The interviewer appears very impressed and pleased with your response.

What do you think will happen? Will you get the job?

Part III

You get a call from one of your friends, who happened to also be on the selection panel. She tells you, strictly off-the-record, that you didn't get the job. She also tells you, strictly off-the-record, that you didn't get the job because of your child.

How do you feel? What might you have done differently? Do you think that will have affected the outcome? What will you do about this (if anything)?

Vignette 14: Bullying (made worse because of your child)

Part I

You have been working at your current job for several years. This is not the ideal place to work from your point of view. The workplace environment is coercive and unpleasant. However, because your daughter is so ill right now and has recently been diagnosed with a serious (and potentially disabling) chronic illness, you believe that your daughter needs your time and attention right now. Your current job is quite close to home, you are confident doing it (and good at it), and it allows you quite a degree of autonomy and flexibility as to when and where you can complete the required work (you often can work from home, or late at night). So you stay.

However, you recently find that you have a new manager. This guy (yes, it is a man) appears to be very nice. He is friendly, appears relaxed and approachable, and has made the appearance of being extremely sensitive about the difficulties you are experiencing right now.

However, when one of the senior managers also asked you about how your child was doing yesterday, at the conclusion of a meeting, you were shocked. You had spoken to your manager in confidence and had told no-one else. He must have taken it upon himself to inform senior management of your situation, without your knowledge or consent.

How do you feel? What (if anything) do you do?

Part II

Over time, while your new manager still appears very friendly and reasonable, you get the distinct impression that he is trying to make your life more difficult. For example, you wanted to break up your upcoming long service leave, taking it in parts, so you could be with your daughter for some upcoming medical treatment. He said that he was 'unable' to help you with this because 'the policy will not allow it'. You check. The policy does allow him such discretion. Why did he lie? Why wouldn't he help? But he seems so nice. Everyone else says he is nice too, and so reasonable. You say nothing about it to anyone.

How are you feeling now? What (if anything) do you do?

Part III

Recently, he has just given you a new project to manage. At first you are flattered. He tells you that you have been chosen because of your particular skill level. You agree happily, looking forward to the challenge. A small voice inside you reminds you that this new role will require longer hours, but you ignore it.

You find however, as you proceed, that the new project is something you know nothing about. Because of your inexperience in this area and because of the previous difficulties associated with this project (for example, a history of complaints from this client), you suspect your manager is setting you up to fail.

He comes into your office, looking concerned, and asks you how your daughter is doing.

How do you feel? What is your response? Why? Would you complain to someone at work? Why or why not?

Notes

Prologue

1 I would like to acknowledge the contribution of Professor Jeff Bailey to the early shaping of this project. It was discussions with him, as well as his contribution to the very early phases of this project, that paved the way for the successful outcomes reported here. I also thank Ms Melissa Parris for her efforts as research assistant.

2 I am delighted to report that, based on the outcomes from the project reported here, I am now leading a much larger, national, Australian study that is focused specifically on the support needs of parents who work full-time and care for a child with a chronic illness. This larger project, commenced early in 2005, will continue for three years and is funded by the Australian Research Council (ARC), the Children's Hospital Education Research Institute, and the University of Western Sydney.

Introduction

1 'Clayton's' is a colloquial term, referring to a nonalcoholic beverage sold and advertised as the 'drink you are having when you are not having a drink'. This term is carefully introduced and explained early in Chapter 6.

Chapter 1   Caring and Working as Work-Home Conflict

1 However, it is also acknowledged that where a child has special needs, such as an intellectual disability, the role of 'parent' may continue well past the age of 18 years.

2 However, while research continues to confirm that women still undertake a disproportionate amount of time with household responsibilities when compared to their partners, it is recognised that, in recent years particularly, married men are beginning to devote more time to household work (Sharpe, Hermsen and Billings, 2002: 79).

Chapter 2   A Useful Research Design

1 For the purposes of this study the term 'chronic illness' is intended to include any long-term, significant illness *or disability*, as defined in Chapter 1.

2 Men were sought but, unfortunately, none were referred for participation.

3 I was not alone in using naturalistic inquiry in combination with other methodological and philosophical approaches. Sullivan-Bolyai et al (2003) used naturalistic inquiry to conduct qualitative interviews and analyse the data from mothers who reported behaviours of constant vigilance to manage the health of their children with Type 1 Diabetes (Sullivan-Bolyai et al, 2003: 21). Zambroski (2003: 32) used naturalistic inquiry to explore the experience of living each day with heart failure, deliberately using purposive sampling to select a diverse collection of participants who shared in common the

experience of living with heart failure (Zambroski, 2003: 33). Baird (2003) also followed this line, in her study of self-care in those with osteoarthritis. Thousand et al (1999) used a Freirean compatible naturalistic inquiry framework known as dialogic retrospection (Thousand et al, 1999: 323) as a research process to elicit voice. Uppermost in all our minds has been hearing their voices to illustrate different themes (Thousand et al, 1999: 323; Vickers, 2005e).

4   Having used Heideggerian phenomenology extensively in the past, I could attest to using all of these in various ways and means (see Vickers, 1998; 1999; 2001a; 2002b).

5   Other studies *have* focused closely on a specific physical or social contextual setting. Belk, Sherry and Wallendorf (1988) used naturalistic inquiry from an ethnographic approach, describing buyer and seller behaviour at a swap meet, a marketing gathering. Mason (2001: 305) used naturalistic inquiry to investigate the learning environment of a class of fourth-graders. Cabaroglu and Roberts (2000: 387) used naturalistic inquiry to explore student teachers' beliefs about language teaching and learning, with researchers being constantly present during a modern languages class at university. Naturalistic inquiry was also used to explore a neighbourhood evaluation, specifically, the post-occupancy evaluation (Churchman and Ginosar, 1999: 267).

6   The project commenced with an additional researcher, who was unable to continue with the project after conducting just two Stage 1 interviews. Unfortunately, it was not possible for those two respondents to continue either.

7   The difficulties experienced in getting respondents to attend the Culminating Group Experience encapsulated the experiences of these women's existence. It was, simply, impossible for most of them to get to any kind of meeting, especially one conducted outside their space and schedule. Despite canvassing the group for possible convenient times, and suggesting possible dates many weeks ahead, just two respondents were able to make it at the appointed time. Others were disappointed, and told me so. They had indicated really wanting to be there – but couldn't. This raised another colourful flag of their existence; too much to do, too little time, and too little available energy, time or space. While I would have liked more to have been able to attend, I did not take it personally nor regard it as negative. I was surprised that any of them could find the time and energy to attend and I remain very grateful to those who did.

Chapter 3   Disconnected and Doing it All

1   It became clear as the interviews progressed that the issue of finding carers was a very important one. Dolly's experience reported here also contributed to the formation of the fictional vignette presented in Chapter 2 (Vignette 10: Childcare concerns) that also stemmed from Cate's experiences.

Chapter 5   Cruelty and Indifference

1   The literature confirms that people assume they must be cheerful and encouraging around sick people (Silver, Wortman and Crofton, 1990: 400) or

those closest to them. However, forced attempts to be cheerful and provide reassurance are often unconvincing, serving only to irritate, or trivialise the situation (Vickers, 1997a; 2001a).

Chapter 6   Clayton's Support

1 The social network refers to persons in a social system that can provide emotional, tangible, and/or informational support (Garwick et al, 1998: 666).

Chapter 7   Working and Caring

1 Sally's views were also represented in Vignette 7 and Vignette 13 (see Appendix).

References

Albelda, R. and Tilly, C. (1998), Glass Ceilings and Bottomless Pits: Women's Work, Women's Poverty, *Working USA*, Vol 1, No 5, pp. 42–55.

Alvesson, M. (2003), Beyond Neopositivists, Romantics and Localists: A Reflective Approach to Interviews in Organizational Research, *Academy of Management Review*, Vol 28, No 1, pp. 13–33.

Amnesty International (1975), *Report on Torture*, Gerald Duckworth & Co, London.

Argyle, M. (1989), *The Social Psychology of Work* (2nd Edn.), Penguin Books, London.

Austin, J. (1990), Assessment of Coping Mechanisms Used by Parents and Children with Chronic Illness, *Maternal Child Nursing*, Vol 15, pp. 98–102.

Australian Bureau of Statistics [ABS] (1998), *Disability, Ageing and Carers: Summary of Findings* (ABS Catalogue No 4430.0), Australian Bureau of Statistics, Canberra.

Australian Bureau of Statistics [ABS] (1999), *Australian Social Trends 1999, Health – Mortality and Morbidity: Asthma* (ABS Catalogue No 4102.0), Australian Bureau of Statistics, Canberra.

Australian Bureau of Statistics [ABS] (2000), *Managing Caring Responsibilities and Paid Employment, New South Wales* (ABS Catalogue No 4903.1), Australian Bureau of Statistics, Canberra.

Australian Bureau of Statistics [ABS] (2001), *National Health Survey: Summary of Results* (ABS Catalogue No 4364.0), Australian Bureau of Statistics, Canberra.

Australian Bureau of Statistics [ABS] (2002), *Health: Disability and Long Term Health Conditions* (ABS Catalogue No 1301.0), Australian Bureau of Statistics, Canberra.

Baird, C. L. (2003), Holding On: Self-Caring with Osteoarthritis, *Journal of Gerontological Nursing*, Vol 29, No 6, pp. 32–39.

Baker, C., Wuest, J. and Stern, P. N. (1992), Method Slurring: The Grounded Theory/Phenomenology Example, *Journal of Advanced Nursing*, Vol 17, No 11, pp. 1355–1360.

Bandura, A. (1990), Selective Activation and Disengagement of Moral Control, *Journal of Social Issues*, Vol 46, pp. 27–46.

Barakat, L. P. and Linney, J. (1992), Children with Physical Handicaps and Their Mothers: The Interrelation of Social Support, Maternal Adjustment and Child Adjustment, *Journal of Pediatric Nursing*, Vol 17, pp. 725–739.

Bar-On, D. (1996), 'Ethical Issues in Biographical Interviews and Analysis', in Josselson, R. (ed.), *The Narrative Study of Lives*, Sage Publications, Thousand Oaks, London, New Delhi, pp. 9–21.

Barnett, D., Clements, M., Kaplan-Estrin, M. and Fialka, J. (2003), Building New Dreams: Supporting Parents' Adaptation to Their Child with Special Needs. *Infants and Young Children*, Vol 16, No 3, July–September, pp. 184–200.

Barron, O. (2002), 'Why Workplace Bullying and Violence are Different: Protecting Employees from Both', in Gill, M., Fisher, B. and Bowie, V. (eds), *Violence at Work: Causes, Patterns and Prevention*, Willan Publishing, Cullompton, Devon, UK, pp. 151–164.

Bateson, M. C. (1989), *Composing A Life: Life as a Work In Progress – The Improvisations of Five Extraordinary Women*, Plume, New York.

Baxter, J. (2000), Barriers to Equality: Men's and Women's Attitudes to Workplace Entitlements in Australia, *Journal of Sociology*, Vol 36, No 1, pp. 12–30.

Belk, R. W., Sherry, J. F. and Wallendorf, M. (1988), A Naturalistic Inquiry into Buyer and Seller Behavior at a Swap Meet, *Journal of Consumer Research*, Vol 14, No 4, pp. 449–470.

Berger, P. L. and Luckmann, T. (1966), *The Social Construction of Reality: A Treatise in the Sociology of Knowledge*, Allen Lane, London.

Bernard, J. R. L. (ed.) (1990), *The Macquaire Encyclopedic Thesaurus: The Book of Words*, The Macquarie Library, Sydney, Australia.

Bianchi, S. M. (2000), Maternal Employment and Time with Children: Dramatic Change or Surprising Continuity?, *Demography*, Vol 37, pp. 401–414.

Bierema, L. L. (1998), A Synthesis of Women's Career Development Issues, *New Directions for Adult and Continuing Education*, Vol 80, pp. 95–103.

Bird, F. B. (1996), *The Muted Conscience*, Quorum Books, Wesport, CT.

Blacher, J., Lopez, S., Shapiro, J. and Fusco, J. (1997), Contributions to Depression in Latina Mothers With and Without Children with Retardation: Implications for Caregiving, *Family Relations*, Vol 46, pp. 325–334.

Blaney, P. H. and Ganellen, R. J. (1990), 'Hardiness and Social Support', in Sarason, B. R., Sarason, I. G. and Pierce, G. R. (eds), *Social Support: An Interactional View*, John Wiley & Sons Inc, A Wiley-Interscience Publication, New York, USA, pp. 297–318.

Blauner, R. (1964), *Alienation and Freedom: The Factory Worker and His Industry*, The University of Chicago Press, Chicago and London.

Bolyard, C. W. (1983), Rescuing the Troubled Employee, *Management World*, Vol 12, No 1, pp. 15–16.

Bonanno, G. A. and Kaltman, S. (2001), The Varieties of Grief Experience, *Clinical Psychology Review*, Vol 21, No 5, pp. 705–734.

Boukydis, C. (1994), The Importance of Parent Networks, Conference Paper presented at the Parent Care Conference, Salt Lake City, UT, 1994.

Bowlby, J. (1946), *Forty-Four Juvenile Thieves*, Bailliere, Tindall and Cox, London.

Bowlby, J. (1980), *Attachment and Loss, Volume III; Loss: Sadness and Depression*, Penguin Books Ltd, London.

Braverman, H. (1994), 'The Degradation of Work', in Clark, H., Chandler, J. and Barry, J. (eds), *Organisation and Identities: Text and Readings in Organisational Behaviour*, Chapman and Hall, London and Glasgow, pp. 385–387.

Breslau, N. and Davis, G. C. (1986), Chronic Stress and Major Depression, *Archives of General Psychiatry*, Vol 43, No 4, pp. 309–314.

Bristol, M. M., Gallagher, J. J. and Schopler, E. (1988), Mothers and Fathers of Young Developmentally Disabled and Nondisabled Boys: Adaptation and Spousal Support, *Developmental Psychology*, Vol 24, pp. 441–451.

Bruce, E. J., Schultz, C. L., Smyrnios, K. X. and Schultz, N. C. (1994), Grieving Related to Development: A Preliminary Comparison of Three Age of Cohorts of Parents of Children with Intellectual Disability, *British Journal of Medical Psychology*, Vol 67, pp. 37–52.

Burgess, D. and Borgida, E. (1999), Who Women Are, Who Women Should Be; Descriptive and Prescriptive Gender Stereotyping in Sex Discrimination, *Psychology, Public Policy and Law*, Vol 5, pp. 665–692.

Burke, S. O., Kauffman, E., Harrison, M. and Wiskin, N. (1999), Assessment of Stressors in Families with a Child who has a Chronic Condition, *The American Journal of Maternal/Child Nursing*, Vol 24, No 2, pp. 98–106.

Cabaroglu, N. and Roberts, J. (2000), Development in Student Teachers' Pre-Existing Beliefs During a 1-Year PGCE Programme, *System*, Vol 28, pp. 387–402.

Campbell, I. (2000), Age and Gender in the Process of Casualisation in Australia, *Journal of Australian Political Economy*, Vol 45, pp. 68–200.

Canam, C. (1993), Common Adaptive Tasks Facing Parents of Children with Chronic Conditions, *Journal of Advanced Nursing*, Vol 18, pp. 46–53.

Caputo, A. A., Brodsky, S. L. and Kemp, S. (2000), Understandings and Experiences of Cruelty: An Exploratory Report, *The Journal of Social Psychology*, Vol 140, No 5, October, pp. 649–660.

Casper, W. J., Martin, J. A., Buffardi, L. C. and Erdwins, C. J. (2002), Work-Family Conflict, Perceived Organizational Support and Organizational Commitment Among Employed Mothers, *Journal of Occupational Health Psychology*, Vol 7, pp. 99–108.

Chambers, M., Ryan, A. A. and Connor, S. L. (2001), Exploring the Emotional Support Needs and Coping Strategies of Family Carers, *Journal of Psychiatric and Mental Health Nursing*, Vol 8, pp. 99–106.

Churchman, A. and Ginosar, O. (1999), A Theoretical Basis for the Post-Occupancy Evaluation of Neighborhoods, *Journal of Environmental Psychology*, Vol 19, pp. 267–276.

Cinamon, R. G. and Rich, Y. (2002), Gender Differences in the Importance of Work and Family Roles: Implications for Work-Family Conflict, *Sex Roles*, Vol 47, pp. 531–541.

Clark, S. C. (2000), Work/Family Border Theory: A New Theory of Work/Family Balance, *Human Relations*, Vol 53, pp. 747–759.

Clark, S. C. (2001), Work Cultures and Work/Family Balance, *Journal of Vocational Behavior*, Vol 58, pp. 348–365.

Cross, A. (1990), *A Trap for Fools*, Ballantine, New York.

Davis, K. (1994), What's in a Voice? Methods and Metaphors, *Feminism and Psychology*, Vol 4, No 3, pp. 353–361.

De Marco, R., Lynch, M. M. and Board, R. (2002), Mothers Who Silence Themselves: A Concept with Clinical Implications for Women Living with HIV/AIDS and their Children, *Journal of Pediatric Nursing*, Vol 17, pp. 89–95.

Dick, B. (2003), Rehabilitating Action Research, *Concepts and Transformation*, Vol 8, No 3, pp. 255–263.

Doty, P., Jackson, M. E. and Crown, W. (1998), The Impact of Female Caregivers' Employment Status on Patterns of Formal and Informal Eldercare, *The Gerontologist*, Vol 38, pp. 331–341.

Drew, N. (1989), The Interviewer's Experience as Data in Phenomenological Research, *Western Journal of Nursing Research*, Vol 11, No 4, pp. 431–439.

Duncan, A. and Miller, C. (2002), The Impact of an Abusive Family Context on Childhood Animal Cruelty and Adult Violence, *Aggression and Violent Behaviour*, Vol 7, No 4, July–August, pp. 365–383.

Dunkel-Schetter, C. and Bennett, T. L. (1990), 'Differentiating the Cognitive and Behavioral Aspects of Social Support', in Sarason, B., Sarason, I. G. and Pierce, G. R. (eds), *Social Support: An Interactional View*, John Wiley & Sons Inc, A Wiley-Interscience Publication, New York, USA, pp. 267–296.

Dutton, D. G., Boyanowsky, E. O. and Bond, M. H. (2005), Extreme Mass Homicide: From Military Massacre to Genocide, *Aggression and Violent Behaviour*, Vol 10, No 4, May–June, pp. 437–473.

Dutton, J. E., Frost, P. J., Worline, M. C., Lilius, J. M. and Kanov, J. M. (2002), Leading in Times of Trauma, *Harvard Business Review*, Vol 80, No 1, pp. 54–61.

Eakes, G. (1995), Chronic Sorrow: The Lived Experience of Parents of Chronically Mentally Ill Children, *Archives of Psychiatric Nursing*, Vol 9, pp. 77–84.

Eagle, B. W., Miles, E. W. and Icenogle, M. L. (1997), Interrole Conflicts and the Permeability of Work and Family Domains: Are There Gender Differences?, *Journal of Vocational Behaviour*, Vol 50, pp. 168–184.

Eagly, A. H. (1987), *Sex Differences in Social Behavior: A Social-Role Interpretation*, Erlbaum, Hillsdale, NJ.

Edwards, J. R. and Rothbard, N. P. (1999), Work and Family Stress and Well-Being: An Examination of Person-Environment Fit in the Work and Family Domains, *Organizational Behavior and Human Decision Processes*, Vol 77, pp. 85–129.

Elvin-Nowak, Y. (1999), The Meaning of Guilt: A Phenomenological Description of Employed Mothers' Experiences of Guilt, *Scandinavian Journal of Psychology*, Vol 40, No 1, pp. 73–83.

Emery, F. (1977), *Futures We Are In*, Martinus Nijhoff Social Sciences Division, Leiden, Netherlands.

Emery, F. and Thorsrud, E. (1975), *Democracy at Work: The Report of the Norwegian Industrial Democracy Program*, Centre for Continuing Education, Australian National University, Canberra, ACT, Australia.

Erikson, K. (1994), *A New Species of Trouble*, W. W. Norton & Company, New York.

Erikson, R. J., Nichols, L. and Ritter, C. (2000), Family Influences on Absenteeism: Testing an Expanded Process Model, *Journal of Vocational Behavior*, Vol 57, pp. 246–272.

Erlandson, D. A., Harris, E. L., Skipper, B. L. and Allen, S. D. (1993), *Doing Naturalistic Inquiry*, Sage Publications, Newbury Park, London, New Delhi.

Eyetsemitan, F. (1998), Stifled Grief in the Workplace, *Death Studies*, Vol 22, No 5, pp. 469–479.

Fabrega, H. J. (1981), 'Concepts of Disease: Logical Features and Social Implications', in Caplan, A. L., Engelhardt, H. T. and McCartney, J. J. (eds), *Concepts of Health and Disease: Interdisciplinary Perspectives*, Addison Wesley Publishing, USA, pp. 485–492.

Farkas, J. I. and Himes, C. L. (1997), The Influence of Caregiving and Employment on the Voluntary Activities of Midlife and Older Women, *Journal of Gerontology*, Vol 52B, No 4, pp. 180–189.

Felson, R.B. (2000), 'A Social Psychological Approach to Interpersonal Aggression', in Van Hasselt, V. B. and Hersen, M. (eds), *Aggression and Violence: An Introductory Text*, Allyn and Bacon, Boston, London, pp. 9–22.

Fenwick, T. (1998), Women Composing Selves, Seeking Authenticity: A Study of Women's Development in the Workplace, *International Journal of Lifelong Education*, Vol 17, No 3, pp. 199–217.

Fine, M. D. (1999), Coordinating Health, Extended Care and Community Support Services: Reforming Aged Care in Australia, *Journal of Aging and Social Policy*, Vol 11, No 1, pp. 67–90.

Fineman, S. (1993a), 'An Emotion Agenda', in Fineman, S. (ed.), *Emotion in Organizations*, Sage Publications, London, Thousand Oaks, New Delhi, pp. 216–230.

Fineman, S. (1993b), 'Organizations as Emotional Arenas', in Fineman, S. (ed.), *Emotion in Organizations*, Sage Publications, London, Thousand Oaks, New Delhi, pp. 9–35.

Fineman, S. (1996), 'Emotion and Organizing', in Clegg, S. R., Hardy, C. and Nord, W. R. (eds), *Handbook of Organization Studies*, Sage Publications, London, Thousand Oaks, New Delhi, pp. 543–564.

Fitzpatrick, R. and Scambler, G. (1984), 'Social Class, Ethnicity and Illness', in Fitzpatrick, R., Hinton, J., Newman, S., Scambler, G. and Thompson, J. (eds), *The Experience of Illness*, Tavistock Publications, London, pp. 54–84.

Florian, V. and Findler, L. (2001), Mental Health and Marital Adaptation Among Mothers of Children with Cerebral Palsy, *American Journal of Orthopsychiatry*, Vol 71, pp. 358–367.

Fricke, W. (2004), 'How to Practice and Train for Action Research: A Non-Positivistic Concept of Social Science', Paper presented at the 20th European Group for Organisation Science (EGOS) Conference, 1–3 July 2004, Llubljana University, Slovenia, pp. 1–8.

Fromm, E. (1942/1960), *Fear of Freedom*, Routledge and Kegan Paul Ltd, London.

Fromm, E. (1963/1994), 'Alienation', in Clark, H., Chandler, J. and Barry, J. (eds), *Organisation and Identities: Text and Readings in Organisational Behaviour*, Chapman and Hall, London, Glasgow, New York, Melbourne, pp. 391–396.

Frost, P. J. (2003), *Toxic Emotions at Work: How Compassionate Managers Handle Pain and Conflict*, Harvard Business School Press, Boston, Massachusetts.

Gabriel, Y. (1998), An Introduction to the Social Psychology of Insults in Organizations, *Human Relations*, Vol 51, No 11, pp. 1329–1354.

Garwick, A. W., Patterson, J. M., Bennett, F. C. and Blum, R. W. (1998), Parents' Perceptions of Helpful vs Unhelpful Types of Support in Managing the Case of Preadolescents With Chronic Conditions, *Archives of Pediatrics and Adolescent Medicine*, Vol 152, No 7, July, pp. 665–671.

Gaymer, J. (1999), Assault Course, *Occupational Health*, Vol 51, No 2, pp. 12–13.

Gergen, M. M. and Gergen, K. J. (1984), 'The Social Construction of Narrative Accounts', in Gergen, K. J. and Gergen, M. M. (eds), *Historical Social Psychology*, Lawrence Erlbaum Associates, Publishers, Hillsdale, New Jersey, pp. 173–189.

Gergen, K. J. (1991), *The Saturated Self: Dilemmas of Identity in Contemporary Life*, Basic Books, A Division of HarperCollins Publishers, Inc., New York, US.

Gibson, C. H. (1995), The Process of Empowerment in Mothers of Chronically Ill Children, *Journal of Advanced Nursing*, Vol 21, pp. 1201–1210.

Gioia, D. A. (1992), Pinto Fires and Personal Ethics: A Script Analysis of Missed Opportunities, *Journal of Business Ethics*, Vol 11, pp. 379–389.

Giordano, F. G. (1995), The Whole Person at Work: An Integrative Vocational Intervention Model for Women's Workplace Issues, *The Journal for Specialists in Group Work*, Vol 20, No 1, pp. 4–13.

Gjerdingen, D., McGovern, P., Bekker, M., Lundberg, U. and Willemsen, T. (2000), Women's Work Roles and their Impact on Health, Well-Being and Career: Comparisons between the United States, Sweden and The Netherlands, *Women & Health*, Vol 31, No 4, pp. 1–20.

Glesne, C. and Peshkin, A. (1992), *Becoming Qualitative Researchers*, Longman, New York.

Goffman, E. (1963), *Stigma: Notes on the Management of Spoiled Identity*, Harmondsworth, Penguin Books, Middlesex, England and Ringwood, Victoria, Australia.

Goffman, E. (1969), *The Presentation of Self in Everyday Life*, Allen Lane, The Penguin Press, London.

Green, P. (2002), 'Naturalistic Inquiry: A Method for Transforming Curiosity into Active Inquiry', in Green, P. (ed.), *Slices of Life: Qualitative Research Snapshots*, Melbourne, Victoria, Australia, RMIT University Press, pp. 3–17.

Greenhaus, J. H. and Beutell, N. J. (1985), Sources of Conflict Between Work and Family Roles, *Academy of Management Review*, Vol 10, No 2, pp. 76–88.

Greenwood, D. J. (2002), Action Research: Unfulfilled Promises and Unmet Challenges, *Concepts and Transformation*, Vol 7, No 2, pp. 117–139.

Gustavsen, B. (2004), Making Knowledge Actionable: From Theoretical Centralism to Distributive Constructivism, *Concepts and Transformation*, Vol 9, No 2, pp. 147–180.

Gutek, B. A. (2001), Women and Paid Work, *Psychology of Women Quarterly*, Vol 25, No 4, pp. 379–393.

Hancock, L. (2002), The Care Crunch: Changing Work, Families and Welfare in Australia, *Critical Social Policy*, Vol 22, No 1, pp. 119–140.

Harris, P., Trezise, J. and Winser, W. N. (2002), Is the Story of My Face?: Intertextual Conflicts During Teacher-Class Interactions Around Texts in Early Grade Classrooms, *Research in the Teaching of English*, Vol 37, No 1, pp. 9–55.

Hastings, D. (1992), 'Adjustment, Coping Resources and Care of the Patient with Multiple Sclerosis', in Miller, J. F. (ed.), *Coping with Chronic Illness: Overcoming Powerlessness*, F. A. Davis Company, Philadelphia, pp. 222–253.

Heilman, M. E. (2001), Description and Prescription: How Gender Stereotypes Prevent Women's Ascent up the Organizational Ladder, *Journal of Social Issues*, Vol 57, No 4, pp. 657–674.

Henderson, S. D., Many, J. E., Wellborn, H. P. and Ward, J. (2002), How Scaffolding Nurtures the Development of Young Children's Literacy Repertoire: Insiders' and Outsiders' Collaborative Understandings, *Reading Research and Instruction*, Vol 41, No 4, pp. 309–330.

Hewlett, S. A. (2002), Executive Women and the Myth of Having It All, *Harvard Business Review*, Vol 80, No 4, pp. 66–73.

Hobfoll, S. E. and Stephens, M. A. P. (1990), 'Social Support During Extreme Stress: Consequences and Intervention', in Sarason, B. R., Sarason, I. G. and Pierce, G. R. (eds), *Social Support: An Interactional View*, John Wiley & Sons Inc, A Wiley-Interscience Publication, New York, USA, pp. 454–481.

Hochschild, A. R. (1983), *The Managed Heart: Commercialization of Human Feeling*, University of California Press, Berkeley, Los Angeles and London.

Hochschild, A. R. (1989), *The Second Shift: Working Parents and the Revolution at Home*, Viking, New York.

Hochschild, A. R. (1997), *The Time Bind: When Work Becomes Home and Home Becomes Work*, Metropolitan Books, New York.

Hodson, R. (1997), Group Relations at Work, *Work and Occupations*, Vol 24, No 4, November, pp. 426–452.

Hopfl, H. (1992), Commitments and Conflicts: Corporate Seduction and Ambivalence in Women Managers, *Women in Management Review*, Vol 7, pp. 9–17.

Hutchinson, M., Vickers, M. H., Jackson, D. and Wilkes, L. (2005a; forthcoming), *'I'm Gonna Do What I Wanna Do'*: Organisational Change as a Vehicle for Bullies, *Health Care Management Review*, October, forthcoming.

Hutchinson, M., Vickers, M. H., Jackson, D. and Wilkes, L. (2005b), *'I'm Gonna Do What I Wanna Do'*: Organisational Change as a Vehicle for Bullying in Nursing, *Proceedings of the 13th International Conference of the Association on Employment Practice and Principles (AEPP)*, 8–10 October, 2005, Baltimore, Maryland, USA, pp. 125–130.

Hutchinson, M., Vickers, M. H., Jackson, D. and Wilkes, L. (2005c; forthcoming), 'Workplace Bullying in Nursing: Towards a More Critical Organisational Perspective', *Nursing Inquiry*, forthcoming.

Ingram, K. M., Jones, D. A., Fass, R. J., Neidig, J. L. and Song, Y. S. (1999), Social Support and Unsupportive Social Interactions: Their Association with Depression Among People Living with HIV, *AIDS Care*, Vol 11, No 3, June, pp. 313–329.

Ingram, K. M., Betz, N. E., Mindes, E. J., Schmitt, M. M. and Smith, N. G. (2001), Unsupportive Responses from Others Concerning a Stressful Life Event: Development of the Unsupportive Social Interactions Inventory, *Journal of Social and Clinical Psychology*, Vol 20, No 2, Summer, pp. 173–207.

Interview Transcripts:
Cate, Interview 1, Tuesday, 15 April 2003.
Charlene, Interview 1, Friday, 25 April 2003.
Dolly, Interview 1, Monday, 7 April 2003.
Dolly, Interview 2, Thursday, 11 September 2003.
Evalyn, Interview 1, Friday, 2 May 2003.
Evalyn, Interview 2, Tuesday, 12 August 2003.
Oitk, Interview 1, Monday, 12 May 2003.
Oitk, Interview 2, Thursday, 4 September 2003.
Polly, Interview 1, Wednesday, 9 July 2003.
Sandra, Interview 1, Friday, 4 April 2003.
Sandra, Interview 2, Thursday, 14 August, 2003.
Sally, Interview 1, Friday, 4 April 2003.
Sally, Interview 2, Friday, 19 September 2003.
Wendy, Interview 1, Tuesday, 10 June 2003.
Wendy, Interview 2, Thursday, 21 August 2003.
Evalyn, Culminating Group Experience (CGE), Thursday, 20 November 2003.
Wendy, Culminating Group Experience (CGE), Thursday, 20 November 2003.

Jack, D. C. (1991), *Silencing the Self*, Harvard University Press, Cambridge, MA.

Jacoby, A. (1994), Felt Versus Enacted Stigma: A Concept Revisited, *Social Science and Medicine*, Vol 38, No 2, pp. 269–274.

James, N. (1993), 'Divisions of Emotional Labour: Disclosure and Cancer', in Fineman, S. (ed.), *Emotion in Organization*, Sage Publications, London, Thousand Oaks, New Delhi, pp. 94–117.

Jena, S. P. K. (1999), Job, Life Satisfaction and Occupational Stress of Women, *Social Science International*, Vol 15, No 1, pp. 75–80.

Jenkins, S. (2004), Restructuring Flexibility: Case Studies of Part-Time Female Workers in Six Workplaces, *Gender, Work and Organization*, Vol 11, No 3, pp. 306–333.

Johnston, C. E. and Marder, L. R. (1994), Parenting the Child with a Chronic Condition: An Emotional Experience, *Pediatric Nursing*, Vol 20, pp. 611–614.

Jourard, S. M. (1971), *The Transparent Self*, Van Nostrand Reinhold Company, New York.

Jutras, S. and Veilleux, F. (1991), Gender Roles and Care Giving to the Elderly: An Empirical Study, *Sex Roles*, Vol 25, No 1/2, pp. 1–18.

Kellert, S. R. and Felthous, A. R. (1985), Childhood Cruelty Towards Animals Among Criminals and Noncriminals, *Human Relations*, Vol 38, pp. 1113–1129.

Kemp, S., Brodsky, S. L. and Caputo, A. A. (1997), How Cruel is a Cat Playing With a Mouse? A Study of People's Assessment of Cruelty, *New Zealand Journal of Psychology*, Vol 26, No 1, pp. 19–24.

Kets de Vries, M. F. R. and Balazs, K. (1997), The Downside of Downsizing, *Human Relations*, Vol 50, No 1, pp. 11–50

Kieffer, C. (1984), Citizen Empowerment: A Developmental Perspective, *Prevention in Human Services*, Vol 3, No 2/3, pp. 9–36.

Kiker, B. E. and Ng, Y. C. (1990), A Simultaneous Equation Model of Spousal Time Allocation, *Social Science Research*, Vol 19, pp. 132–152.

Kinnunen, U. and Mauno, S. (1998), Antecedents and Outcomes of Work-Family Conflict Among Employed Women and Men in Finland, *Human Relations*, Vol 51, No 2, 157–177.

Klama, J. (1988), *Aggression: The Myth of the Beast Within*, John Wiley & Sons, New York.

Kleinman, S. and Copp, M. A. (1993), *Emotions and Fieldwork*, Sage Publications, Newbury Park, California, London, New Delhi.

Knafl, K. A. and Deatrick, J. A. (2002), The Challenge of Normalization for Families of Children with Chronic Conditions, *Pediatric Nursing*, Vol 28, pp. 49–53.

Krieger, S. (1991), *Social Science and the Self: Personal Essays on an Art Form*, Rutgers University Press, New Brunswick, NJ.

Krohn, B. (1998), When Death is Near: Helping Families Cope, *Geriatric Nursing*, Vol 19, No 5, pp. 276–278.

Kubler-Ross, E. (1969), *On Death and Dying*, Tavistock Publications, Sydney.

Kurz, D. (2000), Work-Family Issues of Mothers of Teenage Children, *Qualitative Sociology*, Vol 23, No 4, pp. 435–451.

Laabs, J. (1998), Lottery Workplace Killing Spree Highlights Need for Aggression Management, *Workforce*, Vol 77, No 5, May, pp. 13–14.

Labbe, J. (2005), Ambroise Tardieu: The Man and His Work on Child Mal-treatment a Century Before Kempe, *Child Abuse and Neglect*, Vol 29, No 4, April, pp. 311–324.
La Bier, D. (1986), *Modern Madness: The Emotional Fallout of Success*, Addison-Wesley Publishing Company Inc, Sydney.
Lambert, V. A. and Lambert, C. E. (1979), *The Impact of Physical Illness: And Related Mental Health Concepts*, Prentice-Hall International, New Jersey.
Langan-Fox, J. and Poole, M. E. (1995), Occupational Stress in Australian Business and Professional Women, *Stress Medicine*, Vol 11, No 2, pp. 113–122.
Larrabee, M. J., Weine, S. and Woollcott, P. (2003), 'The Wordless Nothing': Narratives of Trauma and Extremity, *Human Studies*, Vol 26, pp. 353–382.
Larson, E. (1998), Reframing the Meaning of Disability to Families: The Embrace of Paradox, *Social Science & Medicine*, Vol 47, No 7, pp. 865–875.
Lazarus, R. S. and Launier, R. (1978), 'Stress Related Transactions Between Person and Environment', in Pervin, L. A. and Lewis, M. (eds) *Perspectives in International Psychology*, Plenum, New York, pp. 287–327.
Lee, C. (2001), Experiences of Family Caregiving Among Older Australian Women, *Journal of Health Psychology*, Vol 6, pp. 393–404.
Lewis, J. (1995), 'Bullying and School Violence: School Bullies Also Found in Staffrooms', in Healey, K. (ed.), *Conflict Resolution: Issues for the Nineties*, The Spinney Press, Australia, Sydney, p. 31.
Lewis, S. and Lewis, J. (1996), *The Work-Family Challenge: Rethinking Employment*, Sage Publications, London, Thousand Oaks, New Delhi.
Lincoln, Y. S. and Guba, E. G. (1985), *Naturalistic Inquiry*, Sage Publications, Newbury Park, London and New Delhi.
Lukse, M. P. and Vacc, N. A. (1999), Grief, Depression and Coping in Women Undergoing Fertility Treatment, *Obstetrics & Gynecology*, Vol 93, No 2, pp. 245–251.
Mackie, F. (1985), *The Status of Everyday Life: A Sociological Excavation of the Prevailing Framework of Perception*, Routledge & Kegan Paul, London.
Mann, R. (1996), 'Psychological Abuse in the Workplace', in McCarthy, P., Sheehan, M. and Wilkie, W. (eds), *Bullying: From Backyard to Boardroom*, Millennium Books, Beyond Bullying Association, Sydney, pp. 83–92.
Martin, C. and Nisa, M. (1996), Meeting the Needs of Children and Families in Chronic Illness and Disease: The Context of General Practice, Paper presented at the 5th Annual Conference of the Australian Institute of Family Studies, AIFS Conference, 1996, Melbourne, Victoria, Australia.
Marx, K. (1975/1994), 'Alienated Labour', in Clark, H., Chandler, J. and Barry, J. (eds), *Organisation and Identities*, Chapman and Hall, London, pp. 387–391.
Mason, L. (2001), Introducing Talk and Writing for Conceptual Change: A Classroom Study, *Learning and Instruction*, Vol 11, pp. 305–329.
Mattingly, M. J. and Bianchi, S. M. (2003), Gender Differences in the Quantity and Quality of Free Time: The U.S. Experience, *Social Forces*, Vol 81, pp. 999–1030.
Mayhew, C. and Chappell, D. (2001), 'Internal' Violence (or Bullying) and the Health Workforce, Working paper series, in *Taskforce on the Prevention and Management of Violence in the Health Workplace*, Industrial Relations Research Center, University of New South Wales, Sydney, Australia.

McClelland, K. (1985), The Changing Nature of EAP Practice 3, *Personnel Administrator*, Vol 30, pp. 29–37.

McGrath, P. (2001), Identifying Support Issues of Parents of Children with Leukemia, *Cancer Practice*, Vol 9, pp. 198–205.

Mead, M. (ed.) (1955), *Cultural Patterns and Technical Change*, The New American Library, New York.

Melnyk, B. M., Feinstein, N. F., Modenhouer, Z. and Small, L. (2001), Coping in Parents of Children Who are Chronically Ill: Strategies for Assessment and Intervention, *Pediatric Nursing*, Vol 27, pp. 548–558.

Meyerson, D. E. (1994), Interpretations of Stress in Institutions: The Cultural Production of Ambiguity and Burnout, *Administrative Science Quarterly*, Vol 39, December, pp. 628–653.

Miller, C. (2001), Childhood Animal Cruelty and Interpersonal Violence, *Clinical Psychology Review*, Vol 21, No 5, July, pp. 735–749.

Mills, C. W. (1959), *The Sociological Imagination*, Oxford University Press, New York.

Mitchell, T. R., Dowling, P. J., Kabanoff, B. V. and Larson, J. (1988), *People in Organizations*, McGraw Hill, Sydney.

Moen, P. and Elliot, J. (2003), It's About Time: Couples and Careers, *Gender, Work and Organization*, Vol 11, No 4, pp. 591–593.

Moisiewicz, K. (2005), Data Poems in Qualitative Research, Paper presented at the 6th International Interdisciplinary Conference, Advances in Qualitative Methods, February 17–20, Fantasyland Hotel, West Edmonton Mall, Edmonton, Alberta, Canada.

Moriarty, S. (2000), (His) Work and (Her) Family Policies: The Gulf Between Rhetoric and Reality, *Birth Issues*, Vol 9, No 2, pp. 55–59.

Morse, J. M. and Johnson, J. L. (1991), 'Understanding the Illness Experience', in Morse, J. M. and Johnson, J. L. (eds), *The Illness Experience: Dimensions of Suffering*, Sage Publications, Newbury Park, pp. 1–12.

Moss, D. M. and Keen, E. (1981), 'The Nature of Consciousness: The Existential-Phenomenological Approach', in Valle, R. S. and von Eckartsberg, R. (eds), *The Metaphors of Consciousness*, Plenum Press, New York and London, pp. 107–120.

Murray, J. S. (1998), The Lived Experience Of Childhood Cancer: One Sibling's Perspective, *Issues in Comprehensive Pediatric Nursing*, Vol 21, pp. 217–227.

Myers, D. W. (1984), 'The Troubled Employee', in Myers, D. W. (ed.) *Establishing and Building Employee Assistance Programs*, Quorum Books, Westport, CT, pp. 28–41.

Nettleton, S. (1995), *The Sociology of Health and Illness*, Polity Press, Cambridge.

Neuman, J. H. and Baron, R. A. (1997), 'Aggression in the Workplace', in Giacalone, R. A. and Greenberg, J. (eds), *Antisocial Behavior in Organizations*, Sage Publications, Thousand Oaks, London, New Delhi, pp. 37–67.

Newacheck, P. W. (1994), Poverty and Childhood Chronic Illness, *Archives of Pediatric Adolescent Medicine*, Vol 148, pp. 1143–1149.

Noppe, I. C. (2000), Beyond Broken Bonds and Broken Hearts: The Bonding of Theories of Attachment and Grief, *Development Review*, Vol 20, pp. 514–538.

O'Brien, M. E. (2001), Living in a House of Cards: Family Experiences with Long-Term Childhood Technology Dependence, *Journal of Pediatric Nursing*, Vol 16, pp. 13–22.

Oiler, C. (1982), The Phenomenological Approach in Nursing Research, *Nursing Research*, Vol 31, No 3, pp. 178–181.

Oldham, M. and Kleiner, B. H. (1990), Understanding the Nature and Use of Defence Mechanisms in Organisational Life, *Journal of Managerial Psychology*, Vol 5, No 5, pp. i–iv.

Olshansky, S. (1962), Chronic Sorrow: A Response to Having a Mentally Defective Child, *Social Casework*, Vol 43, pp. 190–193.

Osborne, J. W. (1990), Some Basic Existential-Phenomenological Research Methodology for Counsellors, *Canadian Journal of Counselling*, Vol 24, No 2, pp. 79–91.

The Oxford Encyclopedic English Dictionary (2nd Edn.) (1992), Oxford University Press, Oxford, UK.

Page, C. and Meyer, D. (2000), *Applied Research Design for Business and Management*, McGraw Hill, Sydney.

Palshaugen, O. (2004a), Knowledge at Work: New Stories from Action Research, *Concepts and Transformation*, Vol 9, No 2, pp. 113–119.

Palshaugen, O. (2004b), How to Do Things With Words: Towards a Linguistic Turn in Action Research?, *Concepts and Transformation*, Vol 9, No 2, pp. 181–203.

Pavalko, E. K. and Artis, J. E. (1997), Women's Caregiving and Paid Work: Causal Relationships in Late Midlife, *Journal of Gerontology*, Vol 52B, pp. 170–179.

Perrone, J. and Vickers, M. H. (2004), Emotions as Strategic Game in a Hostile Workplace: An Exemplar Case Study, *Employee Responsibilities and Rights Journal*, Special Issue: The Traumatised Worker, Vol 16, No 3, September, pp. 167–178.

Perrons, D. (2003), The New Economy and the Work-Life Balance: Conceptual Explorations and a Case Study of New Media, *Gender, Work and Organization*, Vol 10, No 1, pp. 65–85.

Powell, G. N. (1998), The Abusive Organisation, *Academy of Management Executive*, Vol 12, No 2, pp. 95–96.

Punch, K. F. (1998), *Introduction to Social Research: Quantitative and Qualitative Approaches*, Sage Publications, London, Thousand Oaks, New Delhi.

Quittner, A. L., Di Girolamo, A. M., Michel, M. and Eigen, H. (1992), Parental Response to Cystic Fibrosis: A Contextual Analysis of the Diagnosis Phase, *Journal of Pediatric Psychology*, Vol 17, pp. 683–704.

Randall, P. (1997), *Adult Bullying: Perpetrators and Victims*, Routledge, London and New York.

Raphael, B. (1986), *When Disaster Strikes: A Handbook for the Caring Professions*, Hutchinson, Sydney.

Rasmussen, B. (2004), Between Endless Need and Limited Resources: The Gendered Construction of Greedy Organizations, *Gender, Work and Organization*, Vol 11, No 4, pp. 506–525.

Ray, C. (1992), Positive and Negative Social Support in a Chronic Illness, *Psychology Reports*, Vol 71, No 3, pp. 977–978.

Ray, L. D. (2002), Parenting and Childhood Chronicity: Making Visible the Invisible Work, *Journal of Pediatric Nursing*, Vol 17, pp. 424–438.

Redmond, B. and Richardson, V. (2003), Just Getting on With It: Exploring the Service Needs of Mothers who Care for Young Children with Severe/Profound and Life-Threatening Intellectual Disability, *Journal of Applied Research in Intellectual Disabilities*, Vol 16, pp. 205–218.

Rees, S. (1995), 'Greed and Bullying', in Rees, S. and Rodley, G. (eds) *The Human Costs of Managerialism: Advocating the Recovery of Humanity*, Pluto Press Australia, Sydney, pp. 197–210.

Reiniger, A., Robison, E. and McHugh, M. (1995), Mandated Training of Professionals: A Means for Improving Reporting of Suspected Child Abuse, *Child Abuse and Neglect*, Vol 19, No 1, pp. 63–69.

Renzetti, C. M. and Curran, D. J. (1999), *Women, Men and Society* (4th Edn.), Allyn & Bacon, Massachusetts.

Researcher Notes:

Vickers, M. H., Researcher Reflections, Wednesday, 16 April 2003.

Vickers, M. H., Researcher Reflections, Wednesday, 14 May 2003.

Vickers, M. H., Researcher Reflections, Monday, 9 June 2003.

Vickers, M. H., Researcher Reflections, Thursday, 17 July 2003.

Vickers, M. H., Researcher Reflections, Friday, 15 August 2003.

Vickers, M. H., Researcher Reflections, Monday, 18 August 2003.

Vickers, M. H., Researcher Reflections, Thursday, 16 October 2003.

Vickers, M. H., Researcher Reflections, Monday, 24 November 2003.

Vickers, M. H., Researcher Reflections, Friday, 5 December 2003.

Vickers, M. H., Researcher Reflections, Friday, 6 May 2005.

Vickers, M. H., Researcher Reflections, Monday, 23 May 2005.

Vickers, M. H., Researcher Reflections, Tuesday, 31 May 2005.

Vickers, M. H., Researcher Reflections, Saturday, 11 June 2005.

Vickers, M. H., Researcher Reflections, Thursday, 16 June 2005.

Rest, J. R. (1994), 'Background: Theory and Research', in Rest, J. R. and Narvez, D. (eds), *Moral Development in the Professions: Psychology and Applied Ethics*, Lawrence Erlbaum Associates, Hillsdale, NJ, pp. 1–26.

Robinson, J. P. and Godbey, G. (1999), *Time for Life: The Surprising Ways Americans Use Their Time* (2nd Edn.), Pennsylvania State University Press, Pennsylvania.

Robson, A. L. (1997), Low Birth Weight and Parenting Stress During Early Childhood, *Journal of Pediatric Psychology*, Vol 22, pp. 297–311.

Rolland, J. S. (1987), 'Chronic Illness and the Family: An Overview', in Wright, W. M. and Leahey, M. (eds), *Families and Chronic Illness*, Springhouse, PA, pp. 33–54.

Roskies, E., Louis-Guerin, C. and Fournier, C. (1993), Coping with Job Insecurity: How Does Personality Make a Difference?, *Journal of Organizational Behaviour*, Vol 14, pp. 617–630.

Roxburgh, S. (2002), Racing Through Life: The Distribution of Time Pressures by Roles and Role Resources among Full-Time Workers, *Journal of Family and Economic Issues*, Vol 23, pp. 121–145.

Russell, G. and Bowman, L. (2000), *Work and Family: Current Thinking, Research and Practice*. Report prepared for the Department of Family and Community Services, February, Macquarie Research Limited, Macquarie University, Sydney, Australia.

Rustin, M. (2000), Cruelty, Violence and Murder: Understanding the Criminal Mind, *The British Journal of Criminology*, Vol 40, No 1, Winter, pp. 165–168.

Sandelowski, M. (1994), 'The Proof is in the Pottery: Toward a Poetic for Qualitative Inquiry', in Morse, J. M. (ed.), *Critical Issues in Qualitative Research Methods*, Sage Publications, Thousand Oaks, London, New Delhi, pp. 46–63.

Sarason, B. R., Sarason, I. G. and Pierce, G. R. (1990), 'Traditional Views of Social Support and Their Impact on Assessment', in Sarason, B., Sarason, I. G. and Pierce, G. R. (eds), *Social Support: An Interactional View*, John Wiley & Sons, New York, USA, pp. 9–25.

Sarantakos, S. (1993), *Social Research*, MacMillan Education Australia Pty Ltd, South Melbourne.

Sawyer, M. and Spurrier, N. (1996), Families, Parents and Chronic Childhood Illness, *Family Matters*, Vol 44, No 1, pp. 12–15.

Scambler, G. (1984), 'Perceiving and Coping with Stigmatizing Illness', in Fitzpatrick, R., Hinton, J., Newman, S., Scambler, G. and Thompson, J. (eds), *The Experience of Illness*, Tavistock Publications, London, pp. 203–226.

Schein, V. E. (1993), The Work/Family Interface: Challenging 'Corporate Convenient', *Women in Management Review*, Vol 8, No 1, pp. 22–27.

Schneer, J. A. and Reitman, F. (1995), The Impact of Gender as Managerial Careers Unfold, *Journal of Vocational Behavior*, Vol 47, pp. 290–315.

Scott, D. and Usher, R. (1999), *Researching Education*, Sage, Newbury Park, California.

Seabright, M. A. and Schminke, M. (2002), Immoral Imagination and Revenge in Organizations, *Journal of Business Ethics*, Vol 38, No 1/2, June, pp. 19–31.

Sharpe, D. L., Hermsen, J. M. and Billings, J. (2002), Gender Differences in Use of Alternative Full-time Work Arrangements by Married Workers, *Family and Consumer Sciences Research Journal*, Vol 31, No 1, pp. 78–111.

Shotter, J. (1989), 'Social Accountability and the Social Construction of "You"', in Shotter, J. and Gergen, K. (eds), *Texts of Identity*, Sage Publications, London, pp. 133–151.

Simon, N. B. and Smith, A. (1992), Living with Chronic Pediatric Liver Disease: The Parents' Experience, *Pediatric Nursing*, Vol 18, pp. 453–489.

Silver, R. C., Wortman, C. B. and Crofton, C. (1990), 'The Role of Coping in Support Provision: The Self-Presentational Dilemma of Victims of Life Crises', in Sarason, B. R., Sarason, I. G. and Pierce, G. R. (eds), *Social Support: An Interactional View*, John Wiley & Sons, New York, USA, pp. 397–426.

Smith, R. E. (1979), *The Subtle Revolution*, The Urban Institute, Washington, DC.

Snyder, R. A. (1993), The Glass Ceiling for Women: Things that Don't Cause It and Things that Won't Break It, *Human Resource Development Quarterly*, Vol 4, No 1, Spring, 1993 pp. 97–106.

Steele, C. and Chiarotti, S. (2004), With Everything Exposed: Cruelty in Post-Abortion Care in Rosario, Argentina, *Reproductive Health Matters*, Vol 12, No 24, Supplement, pp. 39–46.

Stein, H. F. (1998), Organizational Euphemism and the Cultural Mystification of Evil, *Administrative Theory and Praxis*, Vol 20, No 3, pp. 346–357.

Stein, H. F. (2001), *Nothing Personal, Just Business: A Guided Journey Into Organizational Darkness*, Quorum Books, Westport, Connecticut, London.

Stevens, M. (1994), Parents Coping with Infants Requiring Home Cardio-respiratory Monitoring, *Journal of Pediatric Nursing*, Vol 9, pp. 2–12.

Stohs, J. H. (1994), Alternative Ethics in Employed Women's Household Labor, *Journal of Family Issues*, Vol 15, pp. 550–561.

Stroebe, M. and Stroebe, W. (1991), Does 'Grief Work' Work?, *Journal of Consulting and Clinical Psychology*, Vol 59, No 3, pp. 479–482.

Sullivan-Bolyai, S., Deatrick, J., Gruppuso, P., Tamborlane, W. and Grey, M. (2003), Constant Vigilance: Mother's Work Parenting Young Children with Type 1 Diabetes, *Journal of Pediatric Nursing*, Vol 18, No 1, pp. 21–29.

Susman, J. (1994), Disability, Stigma and Deviance, *Social Science and Medicine*, Vol 38, No 1, pp. 15–22.

Tal, K. (1996), *Worlds of Hurt: Reading the Literatures of Trauma*, Cambridge University Press, Cambridge and Melbourne.

Taylor, B. (1993), Phenomenology: One Way to Understand Nursing Practice, *International Journal of Nursing Studies*, Vol 30, No 2, pp. 171–179

Terborg, J. R. (1977), Women in Management: A Research Review, *Journal of Applied Psychology*, Vol 62, pp. 647–664.

Thousand, J., Diaz-Greenberg, R., Nevin, A. and Cardelle-Elawar, M. (1999), Perspectives on a Freirean Dialectic to Promote Inclusive Education, *Remedial and Special Education*, Vol 20, No 6, pp. 323–326.

Todd, S. and Jones, S. (2003), 'Mum's the Word!': Maternal Accounts of Dealings with the Professional World, *Journal of Applied Research in Intellectual Disabilities*, Vol 16, pp. 229–244.

Trinca, H. and Fox, C. (2004), *Better than Sex: How a Whole Generation Got Hooked on Work*, Random House Australia, Sydney, New York, Toronto, London, Auckland, Johannesburg.

Turner, B. S. (1987), *Medical Power and Social Knowledge*, Sage Publications, London.

US Department of Labor (1991), *A Report on the Glass Ceiling Initiative*, Office of Information and Public Affairs, Washington DC.

Vallant, S. (2005), Presenting Findings: Creating a Diary to Blend Multiple Stories, Paper presented at the 6th International Interdisciplinary Conference, Advances in Qualitative Methods, February 17–20, Fantasyland Hotel, West Edmonton Mall, Edmonton, Alberta, Canada.

van Eyk, H. (1992), *Caring for Sick Children: How Working Mothers Cope*, Report prepared by the Children's Service Office Consultative Committee, South Australia, for the National Women's Consultative Council, October, Australian Government Publishing Service, Canberra, ACT, Australia.

Van den Heuval, A. (1993a), *Roles Overlap: Workers with Family Responsibilities*. Report prepared by the Australian Institute of Family Studies, Work and Family Unit, Department of Industrial Relations, Australian Institute of Family Studies (AIFS) Monograph No 14.

Van den Heuval, A. (1993b), Missing Work to Care for Sick Children, *Family Matters*, Vol 34, pp. 52–55.

Vickers, M. H. (1997a), *Life and Work with 'Invisible' Chronic Illness (ICI): Authentic Stories of a Passage Through Trauma – A Heideggerian, Hermeneutical, Phenomenological, Multiple-Case, Exploratory Analysis.* Ph.D. Dissertation, University of Western Sydney, Sydney, Australia.

Vickers, M. H. (1997b), Life at Work with 'Invisible' Chronic Illness (ICI): The 'Unseen', Unspoken, Unrecognised Dilemma of Disclosure, *Journal of Workplace Learning*, Vol 9, No 7, pp. 240–252.

Vickers, M. H. (1998), Life at Work with 'Invisible' Chronic Illness (ICI): A Passage of Trauma – Turbulent, Random, Poignant, *Administrative Theory and Praxis*, Vol 20, No 2, pp. 196–218.

Vickers, M. H. (1999), 'Sick Organizations', 'Rabid Managerialism': Work-life Narratives from People with 'Invisible' Chronic Illness, *Public Voices*, Vol 4, No 2, pp. 59–82.

Vickers, M. H. (2000), Stigma, Work and 'Unseen' Illness: A Case and Notes to Enhance Understanding, *Illness, Crisis and Loss*, Vol 8, No 2, pp. 131–151.

Vickers, M. H. (2001a), *Work and Unseen Chronic Illness: Silent Voices*, Routledge, London.

Vickers, M. H. (2001b), Unseen Chronic Illness and Work: Authentic Stories from 'Women in-Between', *Women in Management Review*, Vol 16, No 2, pp. 62–74.

Vickers, M. H. (2001c), Bullying as Unacknowledged Organizational Evil: A Researcher's story, *Employee Responsibilities and Rights Journal*, Vol 13, No 4, 2001 (© 2002), pp. 207–217.

Vickers, M. H. (2002a), Researchers as Storytellers: Writing on the Edge – And Without a Safety Net, *Qualitative Inquiry*, Vol 8, No 5, pp. 608–621.

Vickers, M. H. (2002b), 'People First – Always!': Euphemism and Rhetoric as Troublesome Influences in Organizational Sense-making – A Downsizing Case Study, *Employee Responsibilities and Rights Journal*, Vol 14, No 2/3, pp. 105–118.

Vickers, M. H. and Bailey, J. (2003), Parents, Workers, Carers – And Survivors: A Research Design to Explore Lives and Share Support, *Proceedings of the 5th Australian Industrial and Organisational Psychology Conference, Advancing Creative Solutions in Science and Practice*, June 26–29, 2003, Grand Hyatt, Melbourne, Australia, pp. 39–40.

Vickers, M. H., Bailey, J. G. and Parris, M. A. (2003), Working Parents of Children with Chronic Illness/Disability: Narratives of Concern, *Proceedings of the 11th Annual International Conference of the Association on Employment Practices and Principles (AEPP)*, San Diego, California, USA, 9–11 October 2003, pp. 117–123.

Vickers, M. H. (2004), The Traumatised Worker: A Concern for Employers and Employees, *Employee Responsibilities and Rights Journal*, Vol 16, No 3, pp. 113–116.

Vickers, M., Parris, M. and Bailey, J. (2004), Working Mothers of Children with Chronic Illness: Narratives of Working and Caring, *Australian Journal of Early Childhood*, Special Issue entitled 'Chronic Illness', Vol 29, No 1, pp. 39–44.

Vickers, M. H. and Wilkes, L. (2004), Informal Elder Care and Full Time Work in Australia: A Vital Exploration, *Proceedings of the Twelfth Annual International Conference of the Association on Employment Practices and Principles (AEPP)*, 6–9 October, Fort Lauderdale, Florida, USA, pp. 303–308.

Vickers, M. H. (2005a; forthcoming), Illness, Work and Organisation: Postmodern Perspectives, Antenarratives and Chaos Narratives for the Reinstatement of Voice, *Tamara: Journal of Critical Postmodern Organisation Science*, October 2005, forthcoming.

Vickers, M. H. (2005b; in press), Working and Caring for Children with Chronic Illness: Stories of Disconnection, Cruelty and 'Clayton's Support', *The Review of Disability Studies: An International Journal*, in press.

Vickers, M. H. (2005c), Bounded Grief at Work: Working and Caring for Children with Chronic Illness, *Illness, Crisis and Loss*, Vol 13, No 3, July, pp. 201–218.

Vickers, M. H. (2005d), 'She Hasn't Been Very Well Lately...': Working and Caring for Children with Chronic Illness – Questions of Disclosure, *Proceedings of the Australian and New Zealand Academy of Management (ANZAM) 2005 Conference*, University of Canberra, Canberra, ACT, Australia, 7–10 December 2005.

Vickers, M. H. (2005e), Action Research to Improve the Human Condition: An 'Insider-Outsider', an Emergent Research Design, an Actionable Knowledge Outcome, *The International Journal of Action Research*, Vol 1, No 2, October, pp. 190–218.

Vickers, M. H. and Parris, M. A. (2005), Towards Ending the Silence: Working Women as Carers of Children with Chronic Illness/Disability, *Employee Responsibilities and Rights Journal*, Vol 17, No 2, June, pp. 91–108.

Wallis Consulting (2001), *Victorians' Attitudes Towards Bullying*, Wallis Consulting Group Pty Ltd, Carlton, Victoria.

Watters, J. K. and Biernacki, P. (1989), Targeted Sampling: Options for the Study of Hidden Populations, *Social Problems*, Vol 36, No 4, pp. 416–430.

Wentling, R. M. (1998), Work and Family Issues: Their Impact On Women's Career Development, *New Directions for Adult and Continuing Education*, Vol 80, pp. 15–24.

Werhane, P. (1998), Moral Imagination and the Search for Ethical Decision-Making in Management, *Business Ethics Quarterly*, Ruffin Series: Special Issue, No 1, pp. 75–98.

Werhane, P. (1999), *Moral Imagination and Management Decision Making*, Oxford University Press, New York.

Wilkes, G. A. (ed.) (1979), *Collins Dictionary of the English Language*, Collins Publishers Pty Ltd, Sydney.

Winkler, L. (1981), Chronic Stress of Families of Mentally Retarded Children, *Family Relations*, Vol 30, pp. 281–288.

Wolcott, I. (1993), *Work and Family*, Monograph No 6, Affirmative Action Agency and Work and Family Unit, Australian Institute of Family Studies (AIFS), Sydney, Australian Government Publishing Service, Canberra.

Worden, J. W. (1991), *Grief Counseling and Grief Therapy: A Handbook for the Mental Health Practitioner*, Springer, New York.

Yamada, D. C. (2000), The Phenomenon of 'Workplace Bullying' and the Need for Status-Blind Hostile Work Environment Protection, *Georgetown Law Journal*, Vol 88, No 3, March, pp. 475–536.

Zambroski, C. H. (2003), Qualitative Analysis of Living with Heart Failure, *Heart and Lung*, Vol 32, No 1, pp. 32–40.

Zanetic, S. A. and Jeffery, C. J. (1995), Workplace Communication: The Effect of Gender, *CUPA Journal*, Vol 46, No 4, pp. 13–18.

Index